PLANNING FOR GROWTH AND DEVELOPMENT

PLANNING FOR GROWTH AND DEVELOPMENT

Dr. N. Rajavel

Publications

KALPAZ PUBLICATIONS HOUSE
Delhi–110052

Planning for Growth and Development

Rs. 720

ISBN : 81-7835-514-0

Published in 2006 in India by

Kalpaz Publications
C-30, Satyawati Nagar, Delhi-110052
E-mail : kalpaz@hotmail.com
Website : http://www.gyanbooks.com

Laser Type Setting: Tact Computer Graphics, Delhi

Printed at: Salasar Imaging System, Delhi

CONTENTS

Preface

I am extremely happy and pleased to place this peace of work in the hands of consumers, investors, tourists, development officers, planners for the growth and developments, researchers, students, travel agents, tour operators, organisations, administrations, traders, industrialists, bankers, students, transport owners, entrepreneurs, directors, and officers. This book is the collection of selective writings of the author. He has studied the present burning problems in real sense in the process of the economic development in a systematic way. The author has arrived and suggested the practical solutions to be carried out for such problems and for the growth and development.

For any place, the growth and development fully depend upon the factors around. Such factors are the System of Higher Education adopted, Entrepreneurs, Trade, Commerce and Industry, Consumer Behaviour, Unemployment Problems, Role of Science and Technology, Possibility of curbing the Corruption, Feasibility of Tourism, Tax Reformation, and the Management of Post Tsunami Problems. The growth and development of any area is closely related to the above factors.

Planning is the prime activity of deciding in advance of what to do? What not to do, How to do, when to do? and Who will do? to attain and accomplishment of desired objectives. So all persons involved in the process of growth and development must plan for such growth and development seriously and dedicatively. Hence all are expected to know the basic problem in practice prevailing in the different factorial areas and possible practical and unpainted solutions.

This book covers all the factors involved in the planning of growth and development in five parts namely Part I, Part II, Part III, Part IV and Part V. The Part I is related to the Introduction which covers the framework of this book, Part II consists of Business Related Factors (BRF) viz., consumers, entrepreneurs, trade, commerce and industry and tourism. Part III consists of Education Related Factors (ERF) viz., higher education including examination reformation, science and technology etc., Part IV is fully related to the Problems Related Factors (PRF) viz., corruption, unemployment, tax reforms, and tsunami etc., and Part V is related to the conclusion. Each article has measures to solve the burning problems and suggestions for the growth and development.

This book is written in simple language with the original research work on the current problems. This book will be highly useful to the administrators, government officials, teachers, industrialists, researchers, students, travel agents, tour operators, organisations, administrations, traders, bankers, transport owners, entrepreneurs, directors, officers, head of the organisation and institutions, who are in the process of planning for the growth and development of their own organisation, institution, own projects, units, area, regions, and country or nation as a whole.

I express my sincere thanks and gratitude to all the officers, institutions who have permitted me to visit their units and allowed me to have a frank conversation with their staff. Also I express my hearty thanks to the respondents of my different research work who have very patiently contributed their time in filling up the questionnaires and interview schedule along with their valuable suggestions and criticisms.

I express my hearty thanks to my daughters Miss. Raja. Sudhaa, Miss. Raja. Sangeetha and my son Mr. Raja. Velmurugan for their valuable cooperation in computer typing and correction. I am also indebted to all my friends and well–wishers who extended their help at every stage of the completion of this work. I express my sincere thanks to Mr. Amit Garg, Director Publication, Gyan Publishing Pvt. Ltd., New Delhi for his cooperation in bringing out the book in time.

Dr. N. Rajavel
Port Blair
March, 2006

PART I

1
Introduction

1. Growth and Development

For any region, area or country, social growth, political growth, cultural growth, industrial growth, trade growth and commerce growth are very essential for the development. The economic growth and development forms the basis for the above growths. A country can be said as developing or developed only if it is developing or developed economically. Many authors had given the meaning for the term "Economic Development". Increase in per capita income, coming up of the industrial units, capital formation, full employment, nil poverty, increasing public finance, increasing standard of living are the symptoms of the economic growth and development.

2. Present Scenario

To bring the above symptoms as the situation and status position, every country has been trying their level best since quite a long time. But the result is unsuccessful though not failure. The main reasons for this are poor planning, inefficient organisation, defective communication, baseless direction, system-less functions, less qualified staffing, meaningless control, absence of coordination and careless budgeting.

The people who placed on the responsible position are supposed to plan each and every activity of the system of the management. The drawbacks, failure, carelessness, the quality of taking everything light in the name of positive approach on negative thinkings and happenings, inefficiency, unproductivity on the part of the people on the responsible position, will definitely make the whole investment of funds; investment of energy, productive time, potential hard work and dedicatedness of the efficient people; and the inserted resources etc. to the status of failure along with irrecoverable loss, irrepairable damages, irredeemable investment and unsolvable problems to the country or nation as a whole. In the present day situation that is the people including the controlling officers and the subordinates who are creating problems, committing mistakes, knowing fully that is the Problem and the Mistake. Some instances are:

- Taking Bribe and encouraging the corruption
- Late going to the class and early leaving the classes
- Talking irrelevancies with the students
- Creating the Students' unrest
- Making secret money out of Fund Allocation
- Earning commission from the contracts
- Making policies for disproportionate employment
- Helping and supporting to make false policies
- Using Government Property for self
- Preparing false bills and claims the govt. money
- Seedling indiscipline among the staff and students community
- Introducing dirty politics in the educational institutions
- Criticizing and discontinuing the Dress Codes and effective systems
- Encouraging the sexual relationships among the students
- Encouraging the communal problems
- Encroaching the Government Properties
- Evading Tax and submission of false information to the govt.
- Partiality treatment, harassing the efficient people etc.,
- Willful non-implementation of the Govt. Schemes.
- Fraudulent activities and Misrepresentation
- Using undue influence and so on

3. Planning

So to bring the real growth and development, things are to be decided in advance as: What to do?, What not to do?, Who will do? , When to do? and How to do?. Here deciding in advance means deciding for decision by analysing the pros and cons, merits and demerits, advantages and disadvantages, favourable and adverseness, possible criticisms, benefits and problems. It is not a case, based on thinking something in dreams, compulsion by a group of people having vested interest, and pressure from the political parties, of taking decision and implementing for the result of failure. The quantum of getting success and bringing the meaningful growth and development fully depends upon the extent of effective deciding in advance and taking decision. This is called planning.

So planning plays a vital role in the process of economic growth and development. Once the planning is successful and effective, since it is primacy characterised and featured, the other functions will automatically be formed correctly. Though the management is focused on the environmental factors, the systematic planning can solve the related problems and save the organisation as the ozone layer saves living beings on the earth.

4. Factors

So, by the taking the planning as the basic function for the economic growth and development, the factors and determinants are identified and placed in Three Parts namely Part II, Part III and Part IV. The Part II consists of Business Related Factors (BRF) viz., consumers, entrepreneurs, trade, commerce & industry and tourism. Part III consists of Education Related Factors (ERF) viz., higher education including examination Reformation, Science and Technology etc., and the Part IV is fully related to the Problems Related Factors (PRF) viz., corruption, unemployment, tax reforms, and tsunami etc. They are shown below.

Part-II

BUSINESS RELATED FACTORS (BRF)

1. Consumers

The consumers are the eyes of the business. They are the pillars of the business unit. The ultimate purpose of the production is consumption. Any failure on the part of the consumption will directly affect the growth and development of the business unit. At present situation, the satisfaction to the consumers, conversion of consumers into customers, customer creation, customer retention, consumer based production, consumer based marketing etc. are considered important organs of the business.

There are many says about the consumers. "Consumers are the Finance Providers", "A Satisfied Consumer is the Best Advertiser," "A Dissatisfied Consumer is the Worst Enemy". They are base and foundation of the Economic Growth and Development. So they should not face any problem. What so ever be the planning, the welfare of the consumers is to be taken into consideration by understanding their problems thoroughly.

2. Entrepreneurs

Next to the consumers, the entrepreneurs are very important in the process of the Economic Growth and Development. In fact that "Entrepreneur" is one of the factors of production. Entrepreneur may refer an individual or a group. Entrepreneur is the essence of the business unit because, he bears the risks, combines the other factors and performs the functions, he innovates the new things, undertakes the venture business activities and mixes the 5 Ms.

Fact Afffecting Planning for Growth and Development

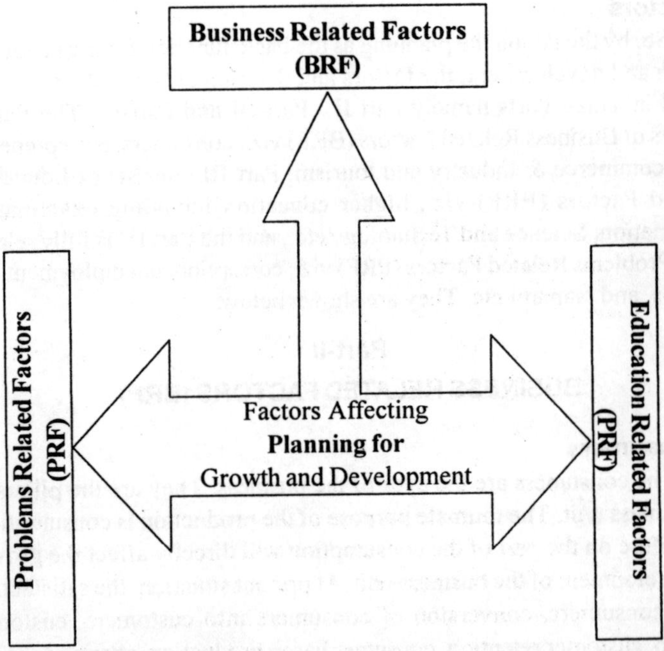

namely Money, Materials, Mechanisms, Men, Machines. He is the person who exploits the available resources, converts them into usable products, reaches them to the consumers, earns profit and gives the share of profit to the government in the name of the tax which is the major source of finance to the government. To be very frank, these entrepreneurs are not given importance in the present days. While planning, this factor of the growth and development has been given very limited importance.

Identification of the true entrepreneurs and encourage them with a view to get revenue for the government from them in the name of tax is the work of the people appointed for the purpose. But once the people get in to the job, they forget the purpose for which they are appointed. How to manage the entrepreneurs and the entrepreneurship qualities efficiently are yet to be understood properly by the related persons. The export of goods and services, earning of foreign exchange, providing standard of living to the domestic population, increasing the domestic income, providing employment, eradicating poverty, exploiting the available resources in a optimistic way etc., are the symptoms of the growth and development for which the entrepreneurs are the main key and they will have play a vital role.

3. Trade, Commerce and Industry

Trade, Commerce and Industry play an important role in the economy of any country. Growth of these sectors is the parameter to measure the economic development in a country particularly developing country like that of India. The contribution of these sectors to the regional development, tax revenue to the government and the national income of the country as a whole is undisputed. Commerce removes the hindrances of person, time, exchange and knowledge in connection with the distribution of goods till they reach the consumers.

Industrial growth, in majority of cases, is the most potent dynamic factor in the process of accelerated economic development. Industry also plays an important role in development backward areas and in removing disparity. Further, the trade, commerce and industry offer ever-widening employment opportunities. Besides generating income and employment opportunities, the development of trade, commerce and industry gives an impetus to social relationships.

4. Tourism

Tourism also is now rightly added to the long list of established industries. Tourism Education is a branch of Business/Commerce Education occupying the status of an Industry. Now Tourism is considered as a part of commerce., Further, as is already pointed out, trade, commerce and industry including Tourism offer ever-widening employment opportunities. Besides generating income and employment opportunities, the development in trade, commerce and industry gives an impetus to social relationships.

Tourism is the Smokeless Industry which attracts the people from different parts of the world and help our country to earn foreign exchange.

Life with Pleasure and live with Pleasure is the recent style of the majority of the people in almost all the countries. In the early days of human civilization, global tourism was not considered as a phenomenon of "pleasure". But in today's world, the tourism on travel has been symbolized as "travel for holiday to get pleasure" and accordingly it has emerged as a way of life. In the past, global tourism was a luxury but today it is available to everyone. Global tourism has two faces namely tourism is a service and tourism as an industry.

Tourism as a service is an old concept and tourism as an industry is newly emerging concept. In general, global tourism has emerged as the most vital and potential phenomenon worldwide and as a result the same has witnessed faster growth rate and has outclassed the world's merchandise exports. Tourism is one of the fastest growing industries in the world. Global tourism as a service and as an industry is a limitless phenomenon with immense growth and development potential.

PART-III

EDUCATION RELATED FACTORS (ERF)

1. Higher Education

Education is a unique future that plays the most dominant role in the life and evaluation of mankind. It is important, as eyes to a man, to his life. A man who is fully educated is the real human resource and is considered as an important, a valuable, and tangible asset to the country. The economic development of the country depends fully upon such real assets. Hence, education – Primary, middle, secondary, higher secondary, college plays a vital role in shaping, sharpening and refining the personality of the person. Higher education provides a proper solution to each problem of human beings, trade, commerce, industry, social, spiritual, culture, political, agriculture, administration, services, and the quality of overall environment. Education, by the curriculum wise, is divided in the Science Education, Technical Education, Arts Education and Commerce Education.

Commerce includes Finance (Banking), Transport, Insurance, Storage, and Advertisement and Publicity. All activities and transactions such as the how to manage, how to prepare accounts, how to bring the relations with the other factors, how to plan, how to organise, how to direct, how to select the personnel, how to control, how to coordinate, how to communicate, how to report and how to budget and estimate etc., related to the Banking, Transport, Insurance, Storage, Advertisements and Publicity are all called commerce activities and the education about such actions and transactions is called Commerce Education which is the basis for the growth and development.

2. Science and Technology

In fact this is the fifth factor of production. It helps the entrepreneurs to go "International". Now a days, the extent and scope of business of the business units do not confined to only internal and they go to competitive global level. For that, they have to find out a lot of new ideas and new products. This is not only for the profit making but also as a responsibility of the business units.

So the entrepreneurs must have the art and science of the business and the activities of the business and management of the units. Innovation is the cover term for the activities of bringing new ideas and invention is the cover term for the activities of bringing something solidly in a physical shape to the world. Both invention and innovations are never ending process and path. So for the economic growth and development, the role of science and technology is very important.

PART-IV

PROBLEMS RELATED FACTORS (PRF)

1. Corruption

In an exclusive definition, the corruption is defined as the "abuse of public office for private gain." It is a plague that attacks our society and economy as a whole. The corruption is the taste of the tasted cat. Now almost the corruption has become a common visible disease. It is very difficult to eradicate but can be tackled to maximum extent. The corruption will create harmful effects to the society.

The corruption may be qualitative and quantitative. Qualitative corruptions are those activities of the corrupts and abuse of the public office for the private gain not in terms of money but in terms of the kinds/ money – able values. Quantitative corruptions are those activities of the corrupts and abuse of the public office for the private gain in terms of money or cash. Of these two corruptions, though these two are dangerous, the qualitative corruptions are more dangerous for the growth and development.

Corruption is very dangerous to not only individuals but also Nation as a whole. Actually, it has to be eradicated completely. But the irresponsibilities of the responsible persons, mismanagement on the part of the managers, carelessness on the part of the officers, uncultured work-culture of the workers and the employees have taken the corruption at present to an answerless question – whether the corruption can be eradicated completely? It has become a normal, now, like a diabetic disease which is almost become a domestic disease.

2. Unemployment

Unemployment is the real problem of a country. It is a social problem. It is very dangerous than the Poison. It is just like an acid thrown skin to the development of the Nation. It is a great threat to the country and its development. It creates inequalities of income, economic imbalance and frustration in the minds of the young educated youth who are going to be the tomorrow's administrators.

The unemployment problem kills the family as a whole. It tempts the unemployed youths (may be of the real human resource) to commit suicides for the want of every day's bread and social prestige. Due to this unemployment problem, the youngsters will be attracted towards the unwanted and anti-national elements. The unemployment problem is a great obstacle to the economic growth and development.

3 Tax Reforms

At present the tax structure is a very complicated with the absence of natural base and justice. At micro level it is, no doubt, one sided. Comparatively the family whose inflow of the cash income more due to the double income pay less tax than that of a family whose inflow of the cash income is less pay more tax. There is an absolute need for the tax reform at this hour and it should continue every year without disturbing the previous announcements.

It is clearly mentioned in the principles of taxation that the Tax Structure/Policy should aim at the increase the resources, reduction of the inequalities, increase the savings and investments and to control the government expenditure. All these principles must be present in the Tax Policy. But the present Tax Structure is not of full-fledged. It lacks some of the important principles. So there is an absolute need for the Tax Reform for the uninterrupted growth and development.

4. Tsunami Problems

Due to the merciless Tsunami, the where–about of the real dedicated teachers, efficient officers, potential youngsters from the different parts of the affected areas are not known till date. The missing list has grown within a short period. The real scene of fighting with Tsunami to save the lives of the children and the people who have escaped narrowly by catching the hands of unfallen trees and thick iron rods are really touching and thrilling. The cries of children and the people who lost their human, physical, tangible and intangible assets are touching the hearts of every living being.

At present, the people of Tsunami affected area are totally in the state of confusion. Once in every day, there is jerking. Sometimes the jerking is intolerably strong which has been increasing the blood pressure of the people and the children. Everybody feels, at present, that they have some sort of giddiness, which is more or less like seasickness at the time of sailing in almost all the places particularly places like Andaman and Nicobar Islands. People fear that the sea level may increase, the seawater may come to their residence and there may be heavy jerking. Almost all the people sleep outside their house during night hours. They are totally worried with confused-state of mind.

As a result, the students do not study, could not concentrate, they fear even to go to their study-room inside the house. The parents fear to send their children to school due to innumerable crackings and less infrastructural facilities to escape from their buildings. This present state of fear is to be totally avoided through a balanced, systematic and corruption-less management of post tsunami problems for the rehabilitation of the people of the affected areas which is the pre requisite of growth and development.

The Selective writings on the each factor or the determinant of the Planning for Growth and Development are given below under each heading.

(I) Consumer

1. A Study of Consumer Problem
2. Role of Consumer Education in Consumer Protection
3. The Consumers and The Need of Their Cooperation

(II) Entreprenurs

1. Role of Entrepreneurship in Solving The Problems of A & N Islands
2. A Study on the Educational Level of the Trade Entrepreneurs
3. An Empirical Analysis of The Educational Levels of Industrial Entrepreneurs
4. Management of Entrepreneurship in Bay Islands

(III) Trade, Commerce and Industry

1. The Toys and Dolls Industry and its Prospects in Bay Islands
2. Manufacturing Industry in A&N Islands – An Analytical Study
3. Role of Banking Industry in The Economic Development of Bay Islands
4. Power and Business Concerns in The Bay Islands

5. Need for Re-Designing The Commerce Education
6. Problems of Industrial Cooperative Units in Bay Islands
7. Management of Cooperative Education and Training In A & N Islands
8. Management of Change.
9. Need For Air Subsidy in The Economic Development of A & N Islands.
10. An Empirical Study on Workings of The Traders in Diglipur Island
11. Management of Traffic Jam

(IV) Tourism

1. Role of Tourism in Economic Changes in Bay Islands
2. Suggestions for Planning Tourism

(V) Higher Education

1. Are We Value Oriented?
2. Need for Reformation in Examination System
3. A Study on Academic Freedom in the Quality of Higher Education.
4. Need For Re-Designing The Commerce Education
5. Management of Cooperative Education and Training in A & N Islands
6. Management of Change.
7. How to Conduct Interview?- A Model

(VI) Science and Technology

1. Concept of Science and Technology in The Economic Development

(VII) Corruption

1. Transparency is a Tool to Tackle Corruption

(VIII) Unemployment

1. White Collared Unemployment
2. Planning a Suitable Career – A Professional Guidance
3. Management of Unemployment Problems
4. How to Conduct Interview?- A Model

(IX) Tax Reforms

1. Management of Tax Reform
2. Need For The Concept of Family Assessment in Tax Reform
3. Computation of Tax Liability of Co-Operative Societies

(X) Tsunami Problems

1. Management of Post Tsunami Problems

I.5. Justification

Of the selected writings, some studies were undertaken by choosing the Andaman and Nicobar Islands as study area. This is because these islands are totally cut off from the Mainland of India. However, these islands are well connected through air service and shipping service. People of these islands face number of problems. Different types of people from different regions, different religions, caste and creed live in Andaman and Nicobar Islands peacefully. The extent of the problems in any part of our country can never be worse than that of the problems facing these islands due to geographical location, less infrastructural facilities and cost of living. So these islands have been taken as the study area for the research work.. Whatever be the suggestions applicable to these islands can very well be tried for any part of our country.

Factors Affecting the Planning for Grwoth and Development

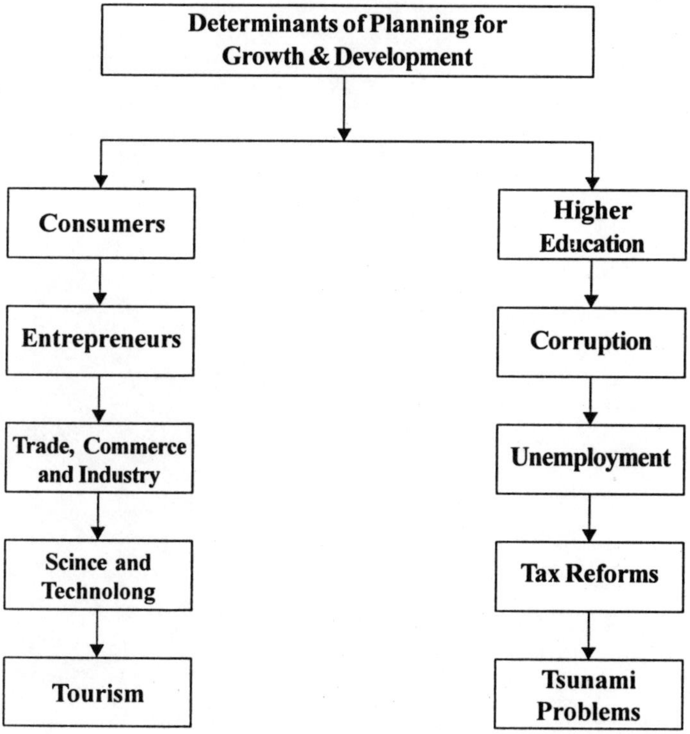

PART II

2

Business Related Factors (BRF)

1. Consumers
2. Entrepreneurs
3. Trade, Commerce and Industry
4. Tourism

Articles...........

1. Consumer

1. A Study of Consumer Problem
2. Role of Consumer Education in Consumer Protection
3. The Consumers and The Need of Their Cooperation

2. Entrepreneurs

1. Role of Entrepreneurship in solving The Problems of A & N Islands.
2. A Study on the Educational Level of the Trade Entrepreneurs.
3. An Empirical Analysis of The Educational Levels of Industrial Entrepreneurs.
4. Management of Entrepreneurship in Bay Islands

3. Trade, Commerce and Industry

1. The Toys and Dolls Industry and its Prospects in Bay Islands.
2. Manufacturing Industry in A & N Islands – An Analytical Study.
3. Role of Banking Industry in The Economic Development of Bay Islands.
4. Power and Business Concerns in The Bay Islands

5. Need For Re-Designing. The Commerce Education
6. Problems of Industrial Cooperative Units in Bay Islands
7. Management of Cooperative Education and Training in A & N Islands
8. Management of Change.
9. Need For Air Subsidy in The Economic Development of A & N Islands.
10. An Empirical Study on Workings of The Traders in Diglipur Islands
11. Management of Traffic Jam

4. Tourism

1. Role of Tourism in Economic Changes in Bay Islands
2. Suggestions for Planning Tourism.

3

A Study On Consumer Problems

Introduction

In consumer education, it is said that the act of production is not complete until the commodity is in the hands of ultimate consumer. It is true that the consumption is the sole purpose of all production. Actually, business is a regular and continuous socio-economic activity to create consumer and to ensure repeat sale which is possible only when the consumers get satisfaction. Consumer-Seller exchange relationship in the market place must be mutually satisfactory. For consumer satisfaction and consumer creation, the business units are fully responsible. In the present dynamic world, every modern business unit has definite responsibilities towards the consumers, the real kings of the business. Whereas, the consumers face a lot of problems in the market due to some business units who do not discharge their responsibilities rightly. Keeping in view the responsibilities of business units as the key point, a study was conducted on consumer problems as no study was conducted earlier in the study area.

Study Area

Port Blair city, the capital of A & N islands, has been taken as Study Area for the present piece of work. Port Blair city has a population of 74,810 as per 1991 census which was 49,634 as per 1981 census. Port Blair city is about 1200 kms away from Madras and Calcutta and is connected through Airways and Seaways. The city offers better prospects for the business activities. The details of the study area and the A & N islands are described somewhere else by the author (Rajavel, 1992)

Methodology

The sample included 120 consumers from the different places of the Study Area. The details of problems faced by the consumers and their opinion about the business units were collected through the Interview Schedule. Twenty selected business units from the city were also interviewed to know their problems and to know the extent of discharging their responsibilities towards the consumers. The data collected were analysed and presented.

Results and Discussions

At the time of interview with the consumers, a lot of problems were elicited from the degree of less importance to high importance. The main and major problems are high-lighted.

1. The consumers often come across artificial shortage called man made scarcities for essential commodities. Huge some of money are used to corner foodstuffs and other essential commodities for the sole purpose of making speculative profits. Business units adopted malpractices of large scale hoarding of many food articles like rice, edible oil, onion, potato, tomato, sugar, kerosene etc. and as a result of which many poor consumers have to pass days without sugar, kerosene etc.. The commodities which went underground are freely available in the blackmarket but at huge price. About 92% of the consumer respondents were of the opinion that the business units are making huge profits. Seventy two respondents representing 60% have expressed about hoarding and black-marketing by the business units and 82 consumers consisting of 68.3% experienced with the adulterated goods. About 76% of the total consumer respondents expressed with heavy heart that the business units of the city are charging unreasonable price.

2. Right to choose, right to be informed etc. are some of the rights of consumers. But as far as the study area is concerned, purchase by choice of commodities is totally absent. Here, the business units dominate the consumers. The person who has been using Hamam soap, Palmolive shampoo, Close-up tooth paste etc. can not continue with the same due to the non availability of such products and hence the consumers are compelled to buy other identical goods at the choice of the business unit. A very important point to be noted is that even in medicines, the consumers of the city have to often go for substitutes. Of the total, 96 respondents representing 80% told that they face a lot of problems due to the absence of choice.

Absence of market information is felt by 37 respondents (30.8%). Forty-two consumers representing 35% have expressed that they were given false representation about the commodities.

3. Short weights and measures are another dangerous problem faced by the consumers. They are not only affected financially but also psychologically. Consumer's hard earned money is simply lost due to this malpractice alone. About 84% of the total respondents stated that they have been facing such problem.

4. Some business units promise the consumers, at the time of sales, that there would be service after sale. But once the sale is over, the units do not give importance to their promise. To confirm the breach of promise, the consumers have to waste their valuable time and money. Thirty-two respondents representing about 26% have expressed the above problem.

5. As far as the business units are concerned, almost all the business units expressed identical problems such as transport problem, finance problem, storage problem etc. but it is observed from the discussion with the business units that no unit bothers about the consumer welfare and the importance of consumer welfare and the importance of consumers. Such behaviour of the units can be viewed in two ways which requires intensive research study at micro level (best area opened by the author to the young researchers). One is, the business units of the city are not aware of the importance of the consumers and their responsibilities towards the consumers and the other is, that they don't want to know the importance of consumers and the responsibilities.

Suggestion

Earning profit is important to every business unit but how to earn such profit is more important than the profit earning. Every business unit has definite responsibilities to the consumers. Each unit should try to retain the customer and should keep in mind that once a consumer always a customer. The following measures are suggested, for the healthy survival of the business units and in-order to remove the consumer problems.

1. Consumers must be given product choices. They should be allowed to exercise their right to choose. They should not be compelled by the business units to buy the substitutes. The business units should allow the consumers to take their own decision.

2. The goods supplied by the business units must meet the needs, tastes and purchasing powers of all classes of consumers particularly of average and common consumers.
3. Sale of goods must be followed by service wherever applicable.
4. Goods must be reasonably priced.
5. Business units must provide adequate and reliable information through salesmanship, advertising, good packaging, labeling etc.
6. Goods must be supplied with correct weights and measures and without any type of adulteration. The business units must give assurance for the quality and service.
7. The consumers should be respected by the business units Consumers may be nervous, dependent, disagreeable, trying, commonsense etc. The business units should deal them very carefully. The units should instruct the salesman not to have any argument with the consumers. They should follow the policy that the consumer is always right.

Conclusion

Consumer satisfaction should be the ultimate aim of every business unit. Now the population of Port Blair city is in increasing trend, comparing the 1981 census the population is increased by about 50% in 1991 census. The sellers cannot have long survival in the market unless they satisfy the consumers by discharging all their responsibilities. Both survival and growth of business depend on consumer satisfaction. So, if the business units discharge their responsibilities by supplying goods with reasonable price, good quality with informative packaging, correct weight and measure, full information, service after sale and without adulterating, hoarding, cornering, false information, profiteering, creating artificial scarcity, the consumer problems will be solved and the consumer-seller exchange relationship in the market place would definitely be mutually satisfactory. Every business unit should remember the following "A Satisfied Consumer is the Best Advertiser and a Dissatisfied Consumer is a worst friend to the Unit".

4

Role of Consumer Education in Consumer Protection

Profit making in any business is not a crime and it is essential for its survival and growth. But illegal profit or profiteering through questionable means like product adulteration, manipulation, fraud, inflating price practices such as hoarding, speculating, black marketing similarly supply of short weights and measures, deceptive packaging, misbranding, unethical advertising and so on are considered as unfair, anti-social and anti-national. The instances and the exploitation through malpractices adopted by businessmen are very long one and hence there is dire need of consumer protection and the consumer education.

Consumer Protection

Consumers are the eyes of the business. They are the kings in the business world. But the importance of the consumer to the business has yet to be realized fully. Business can make profit only when goods are consumed and the services are utilized. Business is entirely dependent on the consumer not only for its very survival but also for its growth. But in real life the consumers are the sufferers of inflation, sometimes controlled or otherwise naked. They pay more and earn much less. They are often cheated through adulterated goods, short weights and measures, deceptive packaging, misleading advertising, hoarding profiteering and other countless frauds. They are to be protected from such malpractices and unfair trade means. Then what is consumer protection? What we need from such protection?

First, we need physical protection of the consumer, for examplc protection against products which are unsafe. Second, we need protection of the consumer against deceptive and unfair trade practices. Consumer must have adequate rights and means of redress against business malpractices and frauds. Third, ecological and environmental effects of chemical, fertilizer or refinery complexes will have to be seriously considered because they pollute water, air and food and endanger human life. Consumer wants due protection against all types of pollution for healthy environment. Fourth, we need adequate protection of consumer against the abuse of monopoly position and restrictive and unfair trade practices. Consumer seeks protection, advise and information when his rights are adversely affected. There are a lot of ways to protect the consumer. Consumer education is one among them.

Consumer Education and Its Objectives

Consumer education means a conscious preparation of the individual in the skills, concepts and understandings that are required for everyday living to achieve, within the frame work of his own values and culture, maximum satisfaction and utilisation of his resources. This consumer education plays a vital role in the consumer protection. It is necessary when numerous consumer goods and services are in the market demanding adequate information regarding safety, performance or correct use of the product. Consumer education and awareness is necessary to bring balanced control among buyers and sellers. It helps the buyer to protect himself against exploitation by unscrupulous sellers indulging in unfair trade practice. It enables the consumers to be aware about the deceptive packaging and misleading labels, tactics of high pressure salesmanship and high powered advertising. A well consumer educated buyer cannot be fooled and cannot be made to pay more than what he has to pay by law. Consumer education gives confidence to the buyer that he cannot be cheated in the market by fraudulent sellers, and essential guidance in learning to detect adulteration of basic foods by simple tests or in spotting out bogus brands of soaps, toiletries, cosmetics, drugs etc. This education can even help families to become aware of their rights and responsibilities as consumers so that they will be able to function more effectively. So the main objectives of the consumer education are

1. to study the consumer, his rights, responsibilities, roles, privileges in the economy
2. to relate the factors influencing consumer behaviour with respect to exchange relationship. That is, the consumer have to be protected from all organisation with which there is an exchange relationship.

Advantages of Consumer Education

The important advantages of the consumer education are as follows:

1. Consumer can achieve competence to live within his income through wise financial management and budgeting.
2. He can achieve competence to determine the best buyers.
3. He will have good bargaining power.
4. He can develop good understanding of market mechanism, market practices and market facilities.
5. He can protect himself considerably against selling frauds and unfair practices.
6. He can exercise his rights of getting information, ventilating grievances and securing their redress.
7. It enables growth of consumer movements speedily as they are aware of their rights, responsibilities etc.
8. It can make consumer protection laws effective in providing legal protection and thereby securing reduction in consumer exploitation.

Consumer Education–Islands' Need

Our A&N Islands is very rich in all resources. But still the market is dominated by the sellers. The consumers of these islands face a lot of problems in the market. So there is a growing realization of the need to educate people at a young age about consumer awareness and to prepare them for the role that they have to play in the economic and social life so that they can make a meaningful contribution to the improvement of their living standards.

Suggestion

In order to strengthen the consumer education, the following suggestions are offered:

1. Articles on important consumer topics, surveys on consumer problems, news and views about the consumer protection and consumer goods may be periodically published through a registered journals atleast quarterly at national level.
2. Talks, seminars and demonstrations may be organized on the consumer protection atleast once in a month in different places of these islands.
3. The above mention two works may be entrusted with the civil supplies department. Moreover, consumer education is closely

related to the commerce education. So the services of the Department of Commerce in the Jawaharlal Nehru Rajkeeya Mahavidhyalaya may be utilized for academic consultations and academic advises.

4. Consumer education may be taken to the classroom where consumers of tomorrow can develop attitudes which will standby them as adult consumers.

5. Consumer education as one of the compulsory papers/ subjects should be introduced in almost all curriculums by all the universities in degree level.

Conslusion

Consumer education is one of the brightest stars on the horizon of business ethics. If the consumer education is given systematically to all the consumers, the consumer will be protected from all such malpractices and unfair trade practices of the sellers. Consumer education is the Consumers' Standard of Living.

5

The Consumers and The Need of Their Cooperation

Intrroduction

In economics, it is said that the act of production is not complete until the commodity is in the hands of the ultimate consumer. In fact, all the production is for consumption either directly or indirectly. It is true that the consumption is the sole end and purpose of all production. Everyone is a consumer, wherever they live, whatever they do irrespective of age, sex, colour or creed. Consumer may be a manufacturer, producer, wholesaler, retailer, gent or dealer. Consumer only, communicate to the producers. "What to be produced" and "What not to be produced". So the consumer is the real King in the free market economy. Without consumers, no businessman can see the profit heaven in the business world.

Consumer Protection

But importance of the consumer to the business has yet to be realised fully. He is the man sufferer of the inflation, sometimes controlled or otherwise naked. Every consumer has been paying more and more but has been earning much less and less in real terms. He is the one often cheated and fleeced – even given shoddy and adultered goods. Of course making profit which will give bread and butter to the businessman, is not a crime but it should not through questionable means like product adulteration, manipulation, fraud, inflationary price practices such as hoarding, speculating, black- marketing, an similarly not through supply of short weights and measures, deceptive packaging, misbranding, unethical advertising etc. These are all considered as both anti- social and anti – national.

So consumer must be protected from those diseases because he has no voice in the product, which is manufactured for his consumption and the majority of the consumers are illiterate and ignorant. Consumer seeks protection, advice and information when his rights are adversely affected. In the year 1962, President John F Kennedy in his consumer message, summed up the rights of consumer and paved the way for organised consumerism in USA and all over the world. The rights of the consumers are:

1. Right to Choose
2. Right to protection of Health and Safety
3. Right to be informed
4. Right to be Heard
5. Right to redress and
6. Right to physical environment that will enhance the quality and quantity of life

In order to protect consumer, the shift from "Buyer Beware" to "Seller Beware" has to be increased and the role of the consumer organisations and Government should be increased.

Consumer Expectations

The prudent businessmen will always look for the consumer satisfaction, which can be obtained

a. By fulfilling their expectations and
b. By treating them nicely and calmly.

Normally the consumers have the following expectations from businessmen.

1. Provisions of wide range of goods to enable consumers to have good choice
2. Supply of goods after cleaning (e.g. grains, spices etc.)
3. Offer exchange facilities if consumer is not satisfied with goods
4. Offer free home delivery to permanent customers
5. Sale on monthly credit
6. Correct weight and measure
7. Reasonable price (uniform price)
8. Unadulterated goods
9. Service after sale
10. Businessmen should not resort to anti- social activities such as hoarding, profiteering, black – marketing etc

11. Frequent supply of goods
12. New design, type, use of goods.

Of course, treating consumers, very nicely and calmly is a very tough job of a businessman. Here only the businessman does see himself. Where he is? What he is? How far he has? Consumers must be convinced. But to convince is not so easy, because the consumers are of different types and nature. They may be nervous, dependent disagreeable, trying and common sense customers. The businessmen must attempt to discover to the customer's feeling and to adjust his goodwill. Types of customer and the businessmen's necessary attempts, in brief, are given below.

Types	*For Customers who are*	*Attempts: Businessmen will need*
Nervous Customers		
	Tired ad Cross	Patience
	Fussy and Nervous	Consideration
	Excitable	Quiet Manner
	Impatient	Despatch
	Unreasonable	Calmness
Dependant Customers		
	Timid and Sensitive	Gentleness
	Undecided	Decisive
	Old and Deaf People	Sympathy
	Children	Power to think for
	Foreigners	Helpfulness
Disagreeable Customers		
	Skeptical	Candid Manner
	Inquisitive	Knowledge
	Talkative	Courteous Brevity
	Insolent	Self Control
Trying Customers		
	Critical	Knowledge of goods
	Indifferent	Tact
	Silent	Perseverance
	Bargain Hunters	Convincing Manner
Common Sense Customer		
	Pleasant	what they expect
	Intelligent	Efficient Service

How to Become a Better Buyer?

To protect himself, the customer or buyer should always be aware of the malpractices. The consumer buyer is an amateur while the seller, by and large, is a professional. So, the buyer must have, while buying the goods, the following guidelines to become a better buyer. Here buyer includes all persons say manufacturers, because he also has to buy raw materials. Wholesalers and Retailers who are the middlemen buying bulk by bulk and by lot and selling by lot by lot and unit by unit respectively, individuals and society at large.

(a) Be prepared about adequate and up- to date information

(b) Avoid impulse buying. Normally average consumer buys in impulse atleast on 50% occasions. The sellers exploit the buyers tendency to purchase impulsively. You should be aware.

(c) Watch for lures and traps, such as bait and switch to deceptive labels etc. bait advertising is used to lure innocent customers into a store. Salesmen may urge you to see and buy more expensive item and the low priced advertised items may not be shown on the sales counters.

(d) Don't believe "get" equals "pay". It is not true that you get what you pay for. There is no close correlation between price and quality. Please be sure that low price will also be associated with higher quality. So go around shopping before buying and justify by comparing the prices, especially in buying costly articles because it can save considerable income.

(e) Read carefully labels, warranties and the date of manufacture or the expiry date particularly in food items and medicines.

(f) In retail trade, retailers would not allow him to be under–sold. You should compel him for price reduction directly or indirectly, for example free house delivery or free installation.

(g) Bargain for lower prices and other concessions or services. You should be more careful when you are going to buy the second hand articles, i.e. say fridge, TV, scooter, motorcycle etc. from your friend because the money – minded friends make use of your gentleness. Don't get or allow to give till the price is fixed.

(h) When you have normal supplies, you can buy in bulk and secure special price concessions in bulk purchase.

(i) Check the quantity; don't be fooled by the size of the package. Label points out net weight, measure, count. Find out whether the package is full or semi – empty.

(j) Check the prices and the total on the bill.

(k) While giving cash and getting balance, cash, count, check and satisfy your self that it is correct. Don't show your dummy and meaningless prestige there. There may be clerical error in calculation and total.

(l) Always adopt cash and carry system. Cash purchases are economical and free from future worries.

(m) Keep records and receipts of purchases. This will help you in replace the product and get quick remedies against your complaints.

Conclusion

In my conclusion, I would like to say that all consumers in order to protect themselves and to come out from the mal practices, should cooperate each other and promote their welfare. The product consumers, manufacturer consumers, wholesaler consumer, retailer consumers and individual consumers, who have been cooperating through "Cooperatives should cooperate more and more to strengthen their cooperatives".

6

Role of Entrepreneurship in Solving the Problems of Andaman and Nicobar Islands

Introduction

The development of any country or region fully depends on the development of economic factors of the country/region. Developing the economy is the only way to break the poverty barrier or the vicious circle and bring into being a self generating economy. The essence of economic development consists in the growth of real per-capita income. Economic progress is the advancement of a community by evolving new and better methods of production, raising the levels of output through the development of human skills and energy, and by acquisition of Capital Resources. Social changes, institutional changes, organisation changes in widespread level are implied in the process of economic development.

Andaman and Nicobar Islands

The Andaman and Nicobar Islands (A & N Islands) situated in the Bay of Bengal and it is located between 60 and 14 of NI, and 92 and 94 of EI. This is surrounded by Burma, Thailand, Malaysia and Indonesia and it constitutes the most isolated part of the Indian Union, stretching in North South direction, separated from Indian mainland by vast stretches of sea. The Andaman Group of Islands are separated from Nicobar Group of Islands by the boisterous 10 channel which is about 155 Kms. Wide and 400 fathoms deep. This territory comprising an area of 8,293 Sq. Kms. is a group of islands. There are 319 islands – 258 islands in Andaman Group and 61 islands in Nicobar Group – in the Union Territory of A&N Islands, only about 38 islands are inhabited. Port Blair, the capital of this Bay Islands, is connected by both sea and air routes with the mainland of

India. The sea distance between Port Blair and Madras in 1190 Kms; between Port Blair and Calcutta is 1225 Kms, and between Port Blair and Vishakapatanam is 1200 Kms. The total population of the territory is 2,77,989-2,38,968 in Andaman District and 39,021 in Nicobar District – as per 1991 Census. This territory is divided into 2 Districts, 3 Divisions, 7 Tehsils and 8 Regions (Rajavel, 1990).

Present Economy of A & N Islands

The economy of A & N Islands, in general, consists of Trade, Commerce and Industry, Forest, Plantation and Agriculture. About 86% of the geographical area is covered by the forests. It is estimated that about 3.63 lakhs Cbm. of different varieties of wood will be available annually on a sustained basis. At present Rubber Plantation, Coconut Plantation, Red Oil Palm Plantation etc. have been taken up in this Bay Islands. Industries in A&N Islands have been divided into 7 categories. There are 339 manufacturing industrial units and 791 trading concerns (R..1990) in A & N Islands. The Commerce of these Islands is divided into 5 types viz. Transport, Banking, Insurance, Storehouse and Advertisement. The islands of this territory are connected by the ferry services and inter-islands Shipping Services. The Shipping Corporation of India and Indian Airlines are operating their vessels between the Mainland at some regular intervals. There are 7 Banks – 6 Commercial Banks and 1 Cooperative Bank with a total number of 37 branches: 3 Insurance Companies (branches) and one commercial Cold Storage in A & N Islands. The commercial activity of advertising is not upto satisfactory level in A & N Islands.

Problems

The Islands of this territory are Economically, Socially, and Politically backward, and are cut-off from the main stream of National Life. So this territory is facing a lot of problems. Increase in Capital Resources, improvement in efficiency of labour, better organisation of production in all spheres, better distribution of goods and services, development of Transport and Communication growth of Banks and other Financial institutions, well constructed store houses including cold storage increase in number of Trading Concerns, improvement in the standard of living are the characteristics of, according to the author, problem free economy. But the economy of A & N Islands is seriously exposed to number of problems. The prices of all goods and the cost of all the services are moving upward trend. The goods which are sold in these islands are not standard in qualities. The customers do not have their choice of goods. They are often compelled to buy the goods which are sold by the traders. In A & N

Islands major potion of resources remain untapped. No proper study has so far been conducted to survey the total available, tapped and untapped resources in the A & N Islands. In this territory, majority of the manufacturing industrial units an wood based units. All consumers durables and capital goods are not manufactured in this territory. So all the goods, raw materials and services are imported from the Mainland of India. For this we can't just blame the traders and industrialists. They face some problems such as, non-availability of space in the transport, extraordinary and undue delay on the part of Govt. official, financial problems, labour problems power problems etc., no body is ready to bear the risks of the business – Trade Commerce and Industry. As far as educational background of the businessmen is concerned, in a survey conducted for the Research work on "Problems and Prospects of Trade, Commerce and Industry in Andaman & Nicobar Islands" (Rajavel, 1990), it is understood that 55.17% of the traders are below matric and only 14.9% are graduates, 66.7% of the industrialists are below matric and only 15.8% are graduates. The reasons responsible for these problems mainly centered around the lack of state initiative in the past, absence of ENTREPRENEURIAL qualities among the existing businessmen and absence of the true entrepreneurs in the A & N Islands.

Entrepreneurships

Entrepreneurs are the kingpins of the business not merely men willing to trade for a profit, but are those who are able to exploit the available resources in the right manner at the right time, a correct outlook training and experience, and in the process create more goods, employment and growth of national income. Till 1800, the concept of entrepreneur was used by the French Economists for adventures, Government contractors, architects, cultivators, those who bought labour and material at uncertain prices and sold the resultant products and contracted prices and those who risked capital in manufacturing. Joseph A. Schumpeter (1934) defined an entrepreneur as one who introduces new production functions. He emphasized innovate aspect more than managerial aspect. To him, a manager remain entrepreneur, only so long as he gives creative and innovative response. According to Francis A. Walker, a true entrepreneur is one who is endowed with more than average capacities in the task of organizing and coordinating the various factors of production. As per the view of Peter Drucker, entrepreneur is one who always searches for change, responds to it, and exploits it as an opportunity. According to him systematic innovation is the fruit of entrepreneurship and the systematic innovation consists in the purposeful and organized search for changes and in the systematic analysis of the opportunities such as change might offer scope for economic or social innovation. So the qualities of a True entrepreneur are:

1. Capacity to assume risk and possessing self-confidence
2. Technological knowledge
3. Alertness to new opportunities
4. Willingness to accept changes and ability to inmate
5. Ability to marshal the resources, and
6. Ability of organisation and administration

Conclusion

In A & N Islands maximum resources remain unexploited. The existing businessmen are only interested in earning money without assuming risks and having the awareness of exploiting the available resources. They really face problems to understand the techniques, principles etc. of the business – trade, commerce and industry – due to their less education. Businessmen of A & N Islands fear to assume risks and hesitate to accept and they lame in in- mataj. Absence of cooperative spirit among the existing traders and industrialists is another problematic feature in the economy of our A&N Islands. As mentioned earlier in any programme of social and economic development of A&N Islands. Cooperative spirit among the businessmen, Govt. officials, Administration as a whole with the people, and the qualities of a true entrepreneur are the Prime requisites. Hence I conclude, the true Entrepreneurial and Cooperative Development programmes only will help in solving the multifarious problems of the area and the people of A&N Islands – viz. Capital loan, Finance, Raw material, Labour, Transport problems, Availability of technical and managerial facility, consumer protection problems etc., to a greater extent because these are the only individuals and organisation which can break the long and solid chain of monopolists (the selfish, interests and corrupt practices) and develop healthy environment for all round development of resourceful A & N Islands.

7

A Study on the Educational Level of the Trade Entrepreneurs in the Bay Islands

Introduction

Trade both internal and international gives a country advantageous to the better industrialisation and standard of living and thereby it increases the economic development of the country. But the Trade and its extent of effectiveness fully depend upon the entrepreneurs the country/region has, the technology they are capable of using, the risk they are prepared to bear, opportunities they are ready to search and accept. The success of an entrepreneur depends fully on the qualities required to innovate, start a new enterprise, accept the challenge and bear the risk. All these qualities are directly related to the education they possess. Trade activities as a whole, is a Sine-quo-non-of economic progress of the Bay Islands (Andaman and Nicobar Islands-A & N Islands). It is one of the important means to improve the economy of these islands. But the growth of Trade in A & N islands is not even at the satisfactory level, though these islands are fully blessed with the resources. Less education or lack of education on the part of the entrepreneurs is one of the main reasons for such slow growth. Keeping in view of trade entrepreneur as the key point, a study has been conducted to analyse the educational background of the present entrepreneurs as no study has been conducted earlier.

Bay Islands

The Bay Islands (A & N Islands) situated in the Bay of Bengal and it is located between 6 degree and 14 degree of NL and 92 degree and 94 degree of EL. This is surrounded by Burma, Thailand, Malaysia and Indonesia and it constitute the most isolated place part of Indian Union, stretching in North South direction, separated from Indian mainland by vast stretches of sea. Andaman group of islands is separated from the Nicobar group of islands by the boisterous 10-degree channel, which is about 155 kms. wide and 400 fathoms deep. This territory comprising an area of 8293 Sq. kms. is a group of islands. Of the total number of islands in this territory, only 38 islands are inhabited. Port Blair, the capital of this union territory, is connected by both sea and air routes with the mainland of India. The sea distance between Port Blair - Chennai; Port Blair -Calcutta and Port Blair- Vishakapatanam is 1190 kms., 1255 kms., and 1200 kms. respectively. The present population of this territory is 2,80,661 as per the census year 1991 and the same will be around 4,00,000 at present as per the projection made by the author. This territory is divided in 2 Districts, 3 Divisions, 7 Tehsils and 8 Regions (Rajavel 1990).

Present Economy of the Bay Islands

The economy of the Bay Islands (A & N islands), in general, consists of Trade, Commerce and Industry, Forest, Plantation, Agriculture and Tourism. Theoretically the forests cover about 86% of the geographical area. At present rubber plantation, coconut plantation, red oil palm plantation etc. have been taken up in this Bay Islands. Industries in these islands have been divided into 7 categories. There are about 400 manufacturing units and about 1000 trading units in these islands. The commerce of these islands is divided into 5 categories namely Finance, Transport, Insurance, Store house and Advertisement. The islands of this territory connected by the ferry services and inter-island Shipping services. As far as the status of the economy of these islands is concerned, it is backward and is cut-off from the main stream of National life. Due to the lack of education and less education on the part of the entrepreneurs in the field of proper exploitation of the resources, all the essential goods, industrial goods, construction goods etc. are brought from the mainland of India. The customers and consumers do not have their choice of goods. They are often compelled to buy the goods, which are sold by the traders who bring goods from the mainland traders. Though a lot of goods and services can be produced and manufactured in this territory itself, they are brought from the mainland of India.

Entrepeneurs

Entrepreneurs are the kingpins of the business not merely men willing to trade for a profit but who are able to exploit the available resources in the right manner, at the right time, and in the process of creation of more goods and employment, and thereby offer a better standard of living to the people of the region. In fact the total population of these islands depends fully on the trade entrepreneurs of this territory. It is not exaggeration to say that the entrepreneurs do business ventures. In the present work of study on the educational level of entrepreneurs is confined only to the entrepreneurs from Trade Sector. The questionnaires have been served only to the trade units. Hence, entrepreneurs in this paper mean only trade entrepreneurs of the A& N Islands.

Methodology

To study the educational levels of the entrepreneurs, a semi-structured questionnaire has been constructed by keeping the education as central point. The questionnaires have been served on a sample of 100 trade entrepreneurs selected for the purpose of this study on random basis. Of the total sample, 91 traders have rightly returned the questionnaires and among these 4 questionnaires were incomplete. Hence, only 87 questionnaires have been taken for the analysation purpose. Besides the questionnaires an informal interview was also held to know their present problem and to know their valuable suggestions. A brief account of the questionnaires is given in Table 1. The results of the analysation and interpretation are given below:

Table 1

Account of Questionnaires

Sl. No.	*No. Particulars*	*Numbers*
1.	Questionnaires served	100
2.	Questionnaire returned	91
3.	Questionnaires rejected	4
4.	Questionnaire taken for analysis	87

Classification

The entrepreneurs are classified to the maximum possible extent. As far as the trade units are concerned the nature of the business is same in almost all the cases. All units buy goods from the mainland and they sell in these islands. So the classification is made on the basis of the forms of business organisation. On the first analysation it is found that the ownership of the trade organisations in the A & N Islands is of four types namely 1. Sole Proprietorship, 2. Partnership firms, 3. Cooperatives and 4. Company. The classification of the sample trade units is given in the table 2.

Table 2

Form of Business (Trade) Organisation

S.No.	*Form*	*No. of Units*	*%*
1.	Sole Proprietorship	54	62.07
2.	Partnership Firms	27	31.03
3.	Cooperatives	5	05.75
4.	Company	1	01.15
	Total	87	100.00

Source: Primary Data- 1999.

The above table clearly pictures that more number of units is in the form of sole proprietorship that is followed by the form of partnership firms. Out of the total respondent units 54 units representing 62.07% are the sole-trader form, 27 representing 31.03% units are partnership form, 5(05.75%) units are cooperative form and only 1(01.15%) unit is company form. This is shown in a diagram Fig.1.

Forms of Trade Business

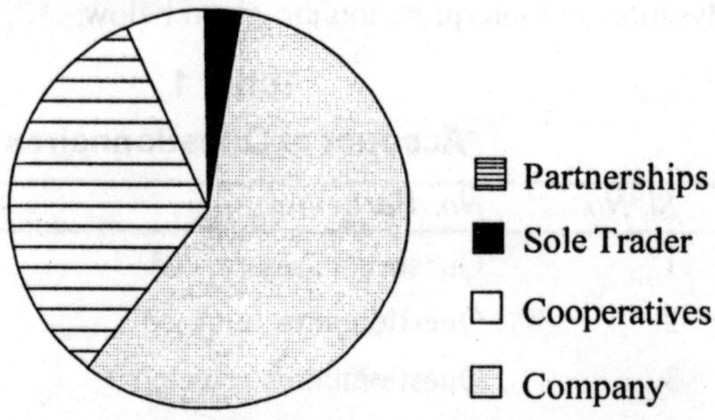

Analysis

The educational qualification plays a vital role in the development of entrepreneurship in the entrepreneurs. As far as the sole proprietorship is concerned, the educational qualification of the owner has been taken;, in case of partnership, the managing partners, and in case of cooperatives and companies the educational qualification of the managing director have been taken for the purpose of this study purpose. The educational qualifications of the trade entrepreneurs as per the information collected through the questionnaires are 1. Below Matric, 2. Matric, 3. Graduation, 4. Post-Graduation and 5. Diploma/Technical. Table 3 shows the number of entrepreneurs with their educational qualifications.

Educational Qualification of the Entrepreneurs

S.No.	*Educational Qualification*	*Number*	*%*
1.	Below Matric	47	54.02
2.	Matric	16	18.39
3.	Graduates	13	14.94
4.	Post-Graduates	7	08.05
5.	Diploma/Technical	4	04.60
	Total	87	100.00

Source: Primary Data-1999.

The table reveals that out of 87 trade entrepreneurs 47 representing 54.02% are below matriculation. Another micro level analysation by taking the form of business organization of the trade units has also been made. Educational levels of the trade entrepreneurs form-wise are given in Table 4.

Table 4

Educational Level of Trade Entrepreneurs on the Basis of Form of Trade Units

Educational Qualifications	*Sole trader*	*Partnership*	*Co-op*	*Company*	*Total*
	No. of Trade Entrepreneurs				
1. Below Matric	32	15	–	–	47
	(59.26)	(55.55)	–	–	(54.02)
2. Matric	11	04	01	–	16
	(20.37)	(14.82)	(20.00)	–	(18.39)
3. Graduate	06	06	01	–	13
	(11.11)	(22.22)	(20.00)	–	(14.94)
4. Post Graduate	04	–	02	01	07
	(7.41)	–	(40.00)	(100.00)	(8.05)
5. Dip/Tech	01	02	01	–	04
	(1.85)	(7.41)	(20.00)	–	(4.60)
Total	54	27	05	01	87
	(100)	(100)	(100)	(100)	(100)

Source: Primary data - 1999.

The above table shows that of the 54 sole proprietorship, 32 units representing 59.26% are managed by the entrepreneurs with the qualification of below matric; 11 units representing 20.37% by the matriculate entrepreneurs; 6 units representing 11.11% by the graduate entrepreneurs; 4 units representing 7.41% by the post graduate entrepreneurs and only one unit (1.85 %) is managed by an entrepreneur with technical qualification. The table also shows that out of 27 partnership units, 15 units (55.55 %) are managed by the below metrics; 4 units (14.82%) by the metrics; 6 units (22.22%) units by the graduates and 2 units(7.41 %) are managed by the technical/diploma holders. No unit is managed by the people with the post graduate qualification. Of the 5 cooperative units, the people with qualification of metric, graduate manage 1 each (20.0%) and technical/diploma holders and the postgraduates manage the rest 2 units (40.0%). As far as the company is concerned, it is (100.0%) is managed by a postgraduate. The table clearly pictures that the entrepreneurs of the trade units are less educated and are need to be educated. Whatever be the experience and other qualities an entrepreneur possess, the less and lack of education and that too commerce education do certainly play an adverse role in the business life. The main reason for such less education on the part of the trade entrepreneurs may be due to the fact that the highly educated persons do not have interest to start a trade/industrial unit but do have interest to go for govt. jobs and the like. It is also understood from the interview with the respondents that they face great difficulties to manage their units due to the want of education and guidance. They depend others (educated) for understanding, drafting, typing and making letters, agreements and contracts etc. Also it is observed from the discussion with the entrepreneurs that they have more working knowledge. Except very few, all are very good in conservation language in Hindi and other limited Indian languages but they face little problem in English language.

Suggestions

The result of the analysation and interpretation of the data collected is that the educational level of the entrepreneurs in these islands is poor. The educational level of the entrepreneurs is to be increased. The following suggestions are offered.

1. At present there is no trade policy in these Bay Islands. A clear-cut and crystal clear Trade Policy and Industrial Policy are to be prepared by bearing the Carrying Capacity, and the available resources of these islands.
2. The existing entrepreneurs of trade units are to be given training, by the local government in their respective branches. The activities of

the initiating agency or agencies if any, may be accelerated to draft suitable project for such training.

3. While preparing the project, the object of the training, need for such training, importance of the training, methodology, procedures etc. are to be discussed in detail by calling the commerce researchers, commerce experts, presidents of the different associations of trade, commerce and industry and the concerned officials. And care must be taken that no politician is to be called.
4. A detailed curriculum for such training is to be constructed. Laws relating trade, commerce, industry, procedure for accounting namely financial accounting, cost accounting, management accounting, office organisation and management, filing system, management of mails, statistics related to the business units, income tax, sales tax calculations, available incentives, subsidies, bounties, concessions etc. are to be included in the curriculum.
5. Local government must take steps to make it compulsory on the part of the entrepreneurs to undergo such training and a clearance from the training institute at the time of applying for the certificate of registration or at the time of renewal of such registration of their trade units.
6. The Government of India must immediately establish an Institute exclusively for the development of Entrepreneurs in these resourceful ever green A & N islands in the grade of Indian Institute of Entrepreneurs. A qualified dedicated person is to be made in-charge of the Proposed Institute.

Conclusion

The different ways and means are to be found out and to be explored to maintain the ecology of these islands and at the same time the industrial and trade activities are to be increased and developed. There are ways and means to develop these islands. The responsible officers must think about the development of these islands. It is very clear from the basic statistics of these islands that the bay islands do not face any financial crises for the development. It is upto the responsible persons to manage effectively. Once an effective strategy is formulated in the light of the suggestions and above discussion and if it is implemented through the real educated, qualified and dedicated persons (not only the officers but also others like academicians) without the involvement of the bureaucrats and politics, and politicians the educational level of the entrepreneurs will increase, and will be increased, and the activities of the Trade, Commerce and Industry shall get accelerated which shall contribute significantly to the overall development of the economy of Andaman and Nicobar Islands.

8

An Empirical Analysis of the Educational Levels of Industrial Entrepreneurs in Andaman and Nicobar Islands

Introduction

Industrialization gives a country advantageous in both internal and international trade and thereby it increases the economic development of the country. But the industrialization and its extent of effectiveness fully depend upon the entrepreneurs the country/region has, the technology they are capable of using, the risk they are prepared to bear, opportunities they are ready to search and accept. The success of an entrepreneur depends fully on the qualities required to innovate, start a new enterprise, accept the challenge and bear the risk. All these qualities are directly related to the education they possess. Industrialization is a Sine- quo non-of economic progress of the Andaman and Nicobar Islands (A & N Islands). It is one of the important means to improve the economy of these islands. But the industrial growth in A & N islands is not at the satisfactory level, though these islands are fully blessed with the resources. Less education or lack of education on the part of the entrepreneurs is one of the main reasons for such slow growth. Keeping in view of the industrial entrepreneur as the key point, a study has been conducted to analyse the educational background of the present entrepreneurs as no study has been conducted earlier.

Andaman & Nicobar Islands

The Andaman and Nicobar Islands (A & N Islands) situated in the Bay of Bengal and it is located between 6 degree and 14 degree of NL and 92 degree and 94 degree of EL. This is surrounded by Burma, Thailand,

Malaysia and Indonesia and it constitute the most isolated place part of Indian Union, stretching in North South direction, separated from Indian mainland by vast stretches of sea. Andaman group of islands is separated from the Nicobar group of islands by the boisterous 10-degree channel, which is about 155 Kms. wide and 400 fathoms deep. This territory comprising an area of 8293 Sq. Kms. is a group of islands. Of the total number of islands in this territory, only 38 islands are inhabited. Port Blair, the capital of this union territory, is connected by both sea and air routes with the mainland of India. The sea distance between Port Blair - Chennai; Port Blair -Calcutta and Port Blair- Vishakapatanam is 1190 Kms., 1255 Kms., and 1200 Kms. respectively. The present population of this territory is 2,80,661 as per the census year 1991 and the same will be around 4,00,000 at present as per the projection made by the author. This territory is divided in 2 Districts, 3 Divisions, 7 Tehsils and 8 Regions (Rajavel 1990).

Present Economy of A & N Islands

The economy of A & N islands, in general, consists of Trade, Commerce and Industry, Forest, Plantation, Agriculture and Tourism. Theoritically the forests cover about 86% of the geographical area. It is estimated that about 3.63 lakhs Cbm. of different varieties of wood will be available annually on a sustained basis. At present rubber plantation, coconut plantation, red oil palm plantation etc. have been taken up in this Bay Islands. Industries in these islands have been divided into 7 categories. There are about 400 manufacturing units and about 1000 trading units in these islands. The commerce of these islands is divided into 5 categories namely Finance, Transport, Insurance, Storehouse and Advertisement. The islands of this territory connected by the ferry services and inter-island Shipping services. As far as the status of the economy of these islands is concerned, it is backward and is cut-off from the main stream of National life. Due to the lack of education and less education on the part of the entrepreneurs in the field of proper exploitation of the resources, all the essential goods, industrial goods, construction goods etc. are brought from the mainland of India. The customers and consumers do not have their choice of goods. They are often compelled to buy the goods, which are sold by the traders who bring goods from the mainland traders. Though a lot of goods and services can be produced and manufactured in this territory itself, they are brought from the mainland of India.

Entrepreneurs

Entrepreneurs are the kingpins of the business not merely men willing to trade for a profit ,but who are able to exploit the available resources in the right manner, at the right time and are in the process of creation of more goods and employment and thereby offer a better standard of living to the people of the region. In the present work of study on the educational level of entrepreneurs is confined only to the entrepreneurs from manufacturing Sector. The questionnaires have been served only to the industrial units. Hence, entrepreneurs in this paper mean only industrial entrepreneurs of the A& N Islands.

Methodology

To study the educational levels of the entrepreneurs, a semi-structured questionnaire has been constructed by keeping the education as central point. The questionnaires have been served on a sample of 75 industrial entrepreneurs selected for the purpose of this study on random basis. Of the total sample, 71 units have rightly returned the questionnaires and among these 8 questionnaires were incomplete. Hence, only 63 questionnaires have been taken for the analysation purpose. Besides the questionnaires an informal interview was held to know their present problem and to know their valuable suggestions. A brief account of the questionnaires is given in Table 1. The results of the analysation and interpretation are given below.

Table 1

Account of Questionnaires

S.No.	*Particulars*	*Numbers*
1.	Questionnaires served	75
2.	Questionnaire returned	68
3.	Questionnaires rejected	5
4.	Questionnaire taken for analysis	63

Classification

The Industrial units are classified to the possible extent. As far as the ownership patter is concerned, of the 63 units, only 07 units are Partnership forms of organisation and the rest are of Sole proprietorship form. Hence the classification has been made on the basis of Raw Materials used. They are 1. Wood Based Units (WBU), 2. Food Based Units (FBU) 3. Sand & Cement Based Units (SCBU), 4. Agro Based Units (ABU), 5. Marine Based Units (MBU), 6. Chemical Based Units (CBU) and 7. Leather Based Units (LBU). This is shown in the Table. 2.

Table 2

Classification of Industrial Units

S.No.	*Type/Classification*	*Number*	*%*
1.	Wood Based Units (WBU)	34	53.9
2.	Food Based Units (FBU)	07	11.1
3.	Sand & Cement Based Units (SCBU)	07	11.1
4.	Agro Based Units (ABU)	03	04.8
5.	Marine Based Units (MBU)	07	11.1
6.	Chemical Based Units (CBU)	04	06.4
7.	Leather Based Units (LBU)	01	01.6
	Total	63	100.0

Source: Primary Data- 1999.

The table clearly pictures that this territory has more number of WB Units that is followed by FB Units, SCB Units, MB Units, CB Units, AB Units and LB Units. Of the total sample units, 53.9% is WB Units. This may be due to the fact that the 86% of the geographical area is covered by forest.

Analysis

The education plays a vital role in the development of entrepreneurship in the entrepreneurs. As far as the sole proprietorship form of industrial organisation is concerned, the educational qualification of the entrepreneurs (owners) and in case of partnership, the qualifications of the managing partner have been taken. The educational qualification of the industrial entrepreneurs as per the information collected through the questionnaires is 1. Below Matric, 2. Matric, 3. Graduation, 4. Post Graduation (P.G), and 5. Diploma/Technical (Dip/Tec). The table 3 shows the number of entrepreneurs with the educational qualification.

Table 3

Educational Qualification of the Entrepreneurs

S.No.	*Educational Qualification*	*Number*	*%*
1.	Below Matric	42	66.7
2.	Matric	08	12.7
3.	Graduates	10	15.8

4.	Post-Graduates	01	01.6
5.	Diploma/Technical	02	03.2
	Total	63	100.0

Source: Primary Data-1999.

The above table shows that the majority of the units are managed by the people whose qualification is below matriculation. Of the 63 respondent entrepreneurs 42 representing 66.7% are below matriculation. This shows that the educational background of the industrial entrepreneurs is extremely poor. Eight representing 12.7% and 10 representing 15.8% of the total respondents are matriculation and graduates respectively. The table also shows that the Post-Graduate and technically qualified people are less interested in starting industrial units. Another micro level analysis by classifying the units on the basis of the raw materials used has also been made. Educational level of the industrial entrepreneurs type-wise is given in Table 4

Table-4

Educational Level of Industrial Entrepreneurs on the Basis of Classification of the Units

Level of Education	*Number of Units*						
	WBU	**FBU**	**SCBU**	**ABU**	**MBU**	**CBU**	**LBU**
1.Below	23	05	07	02	04	01	--
Matric	(67.65)	(71.42)	(100.00)	(66.67)	(57.14)	(25.00)	--
2. Matric	03	01	--	01	02	01	--
	(08.82)	(14.28)		(33.33)	(28.57)	(25.00)	--
3.Graduation	05	01	--	--	01	02	01
	(14.71)	(14.29)	--	--	(14.29)	(50.00)	(100.00)
4. Post	01	--	--	--	--	--	--
Graduation	(02.94)	--	--	--	--	--	--
5.Dip/Tec.	02	--	--	--	--	--	--
	(05.88)	--	--	--	--	--	--
Total	**34**	**07**	**07**	**03**	**07**	**04**	**01**
	(100.00)	**(100.00)**	**(100.00)**	**(100.00)**	**(100.00)**	**(100.00)**	**(100.00)**

Source: Primary Data- 1999.

The Table shows that all levels of education are well represented in the WB Units. Of the 34 WB Units, the entrepreneurs with the qualification of Below Matric manage 23 units representing 67.65%. Five units representing 14.71% with the qualification of Graduation, 01 unit (02.94%) with the qualification of Post-Graduation and 02 units representing 05.88% are managed by the entrepreneurs with the qualification of Diploma/ Technical Qualification.

As far as the FB Units are concerned majority of the entrepreneurs are below matric. About 71.42% of the total FB sample units are managed by the below matrics. All the SCB Units are managed by the below matric entrepreneurs. In the same manner a graduate entrepreneur manages the LB Unit. Two-third of the sample AB Units and one-third of the sample AB Units are managed by the below matrics and matrics respectively. Majority of the educated persons do not have interest to start a trade/industrial unit but do have interest to go for govt. jobs and the like. It is also understood from the interview with the respondents that they face great difficulties to manage their units due to the want of education. They depend others (educated) for understanding, drafting, typing and making letters, agreements and contracts etc. Also it is observed from the discussion with the entrepreneurs that they have more working knowledge. Except very few, all are very good in conversation language in Hindi and other limited Indian languages but they face little problem in English Language.

Suggestions and Conclusion

1. The result of the analysation and interpretation of the data collected is that the educational level of the entrepreneurs in these islands is poor. The educational level of the entrepreneurs is to be increased. The following suggestions are offered.

2. The existing entrepreneurs of industrial units are to be given training, by the local government in their respective branches. The activities of the initiating agency or agencies if any, may be accelerated to draft suitable project for such training.

3. While preparing the project, the object of the training, need for such training, importance of the training, methodology, procedures etc. are to be discussed in detail by calling the commerce researchers, commerce experts, presidents of the different associations of trade, commerce and industry and the concerned officials. And care must be taken that no politician is to be called.

4. A detailed curriculum for such training is to be constructed. Laws relating trade, commerce, industry, procedure for accounting namely

financial accounting, cost accounting, management accounting, office organisation and management, filing system, management of mails, statistics related to the business units, income tax, sales tax calculations, available incentives, subsidies, bounties, concessions etc. are to be included in the curriculum.

5. Local government must take steps to make it compulsory on the part of the entrepreneurs to undergo such training and a clearance from the training institute at the time of applying for the certificate of registration or at the time of renewal of such registration of their industrial units.

6. The Government of India must immediately establish an Institute exclusively for the development of Entrepreneurs in these resourceful evergreen A & N islands in the grade of Indian Institute of Entrepreneurs. A qualified dedicated person is to be made in-charge of the Proposed Institute.

Once an effective strategy is formulated in the light of the suggestions and above discussion and if it is implemented through the real educated, qualified and dedicated academicians without the involvement of the bureaucrats and politics, the educational level of the entrepreneurs will increase, and will be increased, and the activities of the Trade, Commerce and Industry shall get accelerated which shall contribute significantly to the overall development of the Economy of Andaman and Nicobar Islands.

9

Management of Entrepreneurship in Bay Islands

Introduction

At any particular moment of time, any economy has a certain maximum potential rate of growth. This depends on the entrepreneurs it has, the technology they are capable of using, the amount they are prepared to invest, and the various bottlenecks which would check an upward movement at a faster pace, such as scarcity of skilled labour or the various scarcities of equipments and war materials which translate into scarcity foreign exchange. If anyone wishes to move the economy faster, he/she must understand the factors influencing the Entrepreneurship in entrepreneurs in entrepreneurs' development. Since the author wants that every one of us must wish to move the economy of Andaman & Nicobar Islands (Bay Islands) faster, this paper is presented on the need for the Entrepreneurial development in Bay Islands.

Andaman & Nicobar Islands and Its Economy

Andaman & Nicobar Islands is situated in the Bay of Bengal and it is located between the 6 degree and 4 degree NL and 92 degree and 94 degree EL. Burma, Thailand, Malaysia and Indonesia surround this island and it constitutes the most isolated part of the Indian Union. This territory, comprising an area of 8,293 sq. kms., is a group of picturesque islands. Port Blair is the capital and the only city of this Bay Islands, is connected with the mainland of India by both the air routes and sea. The total population of this territory is 2,80,661 as per 1991 census. The economy of Andaman & Nicobar Islands is constituted by agricultural sector, industrial sector and trading sector. Of these three sectors, Industrial sector has an excellent scope for its development in this territory is still in infant stage.

Entreprenuership

Entrepreneurs play a central role in the process of industrial development of these islands. Entrepreneurial competence or the Entrepreneurship is a key ingredient of which industrial development can be achieved in this territory. Entrepreneurship means, in the words of Higgins, "the function of seeking investment and production opportunity, organising and enterprise to undertake a new production process, raising capital , hiring labour, arranging the supply raw material, finding site, introducing new techniques and commodities, discovering new sources of raw materials and selecting top managers from day to day operations of the enterprise." That means, the capacity to take or assume risks, i.e., make an investment decisions under the condition of uncertainty, capacity to plan, capacity to innovate and the capacity to take prompt and sound decisions concerning production and marketing are necessary qualities of an entrepreneurs. It is felt that inadequate availability of entrepreneurial talent in these islands appears to be main reason for the low level of industrial development in this territory.

Influencing Factors

The qualities, capacities and capabilities in the entrepreneurs should be increased. Entrepreneurship is a function of certain socio- economic and cultural setting. In order to develop, the Entrepreneurship in the islands, one should take into account and understand the economic condition of individuals, the culture and the society of the Bay islands. The following factors are influencing the entrepreneurial development in these islands.

- Resources
- Raw materials
- Organizations that stimulate and provide institutional support
- Infrastructural facilities
- The entrepreneurs

Management

I am very proud to say, what is not in Andaman & Nicobar Islands. This territory is very rich in her resources. Natural resources, agricultural resources, forest resources, human resources, plantation resources are plenty in Andaman & Nicobar Islands but unutilized and unexploited. Abundant human resources available in this territory but. It they are untrained and unskilled. There are various institutions and organizations for providing institutional support to the entrepreneurs but their functioning is not upto satisfactory level and not proper. There is acute problem of infrastructural facilities in this territory and this is more acute in other islands. But the entrepreneurs are more in the Andaman & Nicobar Islands in front of entrepreneurial talents. To be more specific, the author wants to point out that our territory is also having sorts of resources, different organizations in order to supports the entrepreneurs but the industrial development is still infant stage and did not make any markable contribution to the national income of the Andaman & Nicobar Islands. Therefore, we need a concrete action programme for the entrepreneurial development in these islands. Such programme may be undertaken in the following stages.

1. Intensive advertisement and publicity
2. Stimulation
3. Delay avoidance
4. Orientation
5. Technical guidance
6. Promotion
7. Follow up

Management

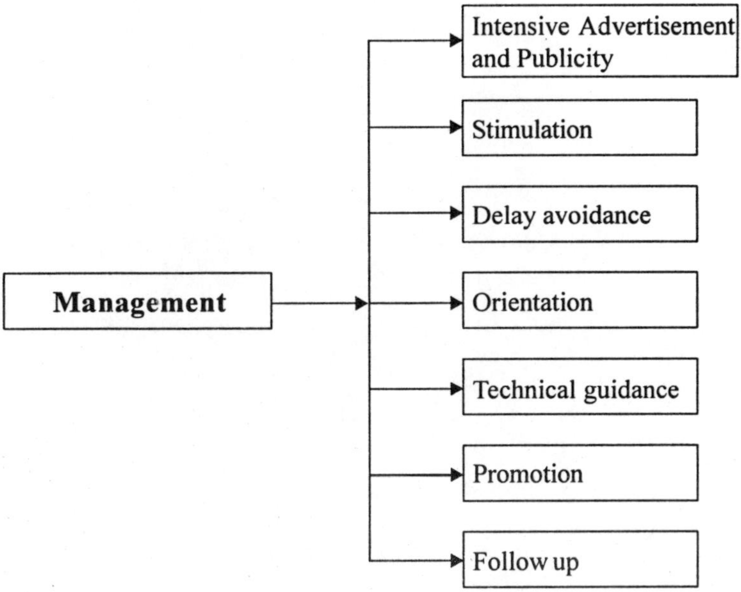

Suggestions

Among the above mentioned seven stages, identifications and follow up are very important. There must be sincere and carefulness in identification and continuity in follow up. All locally available resources must be gradually and fully utilized and exploited. Proper and sincere training facilities must be given to the entrepreneurs. The life killing undue delay in approvals, sanctions, connections, and the likes etc. should be totally avoided. The Officers turn over must be kept as minimum as possible.

Conclusion

I would like to conclude that every one of us must sincerely think to move the economy of Andaman & Nicobar Islands faster. If a concrete programme in the light of the above discussions with the above-mentioned stages is constructed, I am very sure that the entrepreneurial development in Bay islands will increase and the economy of the Andaman & Nicobar Islands will move faster.

10

The Toys and Dolls Industry and Its Prospects in Bay Islands

Abstract

The present paper deals with prospects of Toys and Dolls Industry in the Bay Islands. After emphasizing the availability of raw materials, present status of the industry, problems involved in setting new units are discussed in detail. The guidelines to promote the industry at administrative, finance, power, marketing and export levels are suggested.

Introduction

The Government of India has been emphasizing the industrialization of the country with a view to create employment, to increase export and to raise production and productivity for over all development of the economy. Toys and Dolls Industry is also one of the industries which is contributing its major share in the world market besides catering mainly to the requirements of the domestic market. But in the Andaman and Nicobar Islands there is no such industry or unit manufacturing Toys and Dolls inspite of the availability of raw materials in abundance and the suitable industrial climate. Moreover, no study has been conducted so far about this industry in these islands. Hence, an attempt has been made in this paper to study the industrial climate, market potential for Toys and Dolls, prospects of Toys and Dolls Industry, available resources and anticipated problems of the industry.

The Study Area

The Andaman and Nicobar Islands situated in the Bay of Bengal are surrounded by Burma, Thailand, Malaysia and Indonesia. The Islands constitute the most isolated part of the Indian Union, stretching in North-

South direction, separated from Indian mainland by vast stretches of sea. The Andaman group of islands are separated from the Nicobar group of islands by the boisterous 10° channel which is about 155 Kms. Wide and 400 fathoms deep. This territory, comprising an area of 8,293 Sq. Kms., is a group of picturesque islands. There are 258 islands in the Andaman group and 61 islands in the Nicobar group. Only about 38 islands are inhabited. Port Blair, the capital of this Bay Islands, is connected with the mainland by both sea and air routes. The sea distance between Port Blair and Madras is 1,190 Kms., between Port Blair and Calcutta is 1,255 Kms., and between Port Blair and Vishakapatanam is 1,200 Kms. The total population of these islands is 2,77,989; 2,38,968 in Andaman District and 39,021 in Nicobar District – as per 1991 census. This territory is divided into 2 Districts, 3 Divisions 7 Tehsils and 8 Regions (Rajavel,1990) as shown in Table No.1.

Methodology

This study has been undertaken to trace the market potentially for Toys and Dolls to visualize the available resources and industrial climate, to bring out the prospects and future problems, and to offer suitable suggestions to establish the industry. In this regard, mainly secondary data have been taken. The traders dealing in Toys and Dolls, the industrialists (village units) who are manufacturing Dolls (mono style) out of timber, and some interested entrepreneurs in these islands and existing Toys and Dolls makers in the Districts of South Arcot, Thanjavur and Thiruchirapalli of Tamil Nadu State were interviewed informally. The author personally visited the factories in the mainland to know the processes, designs, models, etc.

Industrial Climate

The Union territory of Andaman and Nicobar Islands is industrially very backward. In the whole territory, the Nicobar District has been declared as, 'No Industry Area'. Till 1978, there was no full-fledged industries Department in this territory. Only in March, 1978, the Directorate of Industries and the District Industries Centre were set up. They are promoting few units every year. Industries in the Andaman & Nicobar islands are divided into 7 categories (Rajavel,1990). They are Wood Based Industry, Food Based Industry, Marine Based Industry, Agro Based Industry, Chemical Based Industry and Leather Based Industry is the biggest industry in the Andaman and Nicobar Islands.

There are 187 units under this industry. The units manufacturing furniture, plywood, pencil slates, match splints and dolls (mono style) etc. constitute the Wood Based Industry. But there is no Toy making unit in the Andaman and Nicobar Islands. Even in the Chemical Based Industry, there is no such unit. Taking the total number of units under the Wood Based Industry, except 24 units-6 medium scale and 18 small scale units-out of the 187 units almost all the units manufacture Dancing Dolls out of the superior quality wood named Padak. Dancing Dolls are manufactured on monotype model. There is no other model of Dolls in any raw material manufactured in this factory.

Market Potentialities

Toys and Dolls making industry, in India, is essentially a village and cottage industry. But in the Andaman and Nicobar Islands, though there are considerable prospects and resources, and market potentialities, there is no Toy making unit. The absence of and the presence of potentialities and prospects for, this industry in this territory inspires the author to conduct a micro level study on the scope for Toys and Dolls Industry in this territory.

The Andaman and Nicobar Islands has a great potential to manufacture Toys and Dolls and market the same both in the local, mainland and foreign markets. There is a growing market for the dancing dolls in the Andaman and Nicobar Islands. Almost in all the houses the dancing dolls are kept as a beauty article. Tourists, both Indian and foreign, are attracted by these dancing dolls. So there is a sales outlet for the dancing doll both at the harbour on ship days and at the airport on all flight days. Tourists purchase on an average of 2-4 dolls per family from the different small units, and shops at bazaars or sales outlets at the harbour and at the airport. The author witnessed many times that these dancing dolls are presented on the occasions like marriages, birthdays etc. in the mainland with the goodwill of "a gift from Andaman and Nicobar Islands". The price of the dolls varies according to the size. The price ranges from Rs. 40/- to Rs. 500/-. An interesting point to be noted is that the price of a female image doll is always higher than the price of the male image doll. Increasing demand for the wooden dolls is the evidence for the good prospects for the Toys and Dolls Industry in the Bay Islands.

Prospects

The dolls manufactured in the Andaman and Nicobar Islands are of the same style and model. Considerable change in style, model and size has to be made. This will increase the demand for the products. Talking Dolls, Musical Dolls, Walking Dolls, and Dolls with other actions, are to be introduced and manufactured. As far as the size of the Dolls is concerned, all sizes should be made available. This will facilitate all agars to purchase the dolls. For example very small size will be used for children to play and the big size will be used to put as show piece in houses, offices, etc. so far no manufacturer has manufactured Live Size Baby Doll. It is forecast that there will be huge demand for the Live Size Baby Doll, both in the markets of local, mainland and abroad. One more important feature to be noted is that there is no specialized shop for doll business in the territory.

As far as Toys are concerned, as is mentioned earlier, there is no toy making industry in the Andaman and Nicobar Islands. Only limited number of shops in Port Blair Region, Rangat Region, Mayabunder Region, Diglipur Region and Campbell Bay Region are selling toys made out of rubber and plastics as one of the items in the shops. Toys are very popular with the children of the age group of 10 years and below. Trade Development Authority of India has conducted a contact promotion programme for Toys and Dolls in UK, FRG and France. They found the product requirements according to the age group in these countries which is given in Table No. 2. This is almost true in our country also. This age group consists of about 75 thousands i.e. about 25% of the total population in the Andaman and Nicobar Islands. Although all types of toys are in demand, yet it is observed that the demand for electronic toys is increasing steadily. The plastic toys, rubber toys and wooden toys are imported from the mainland of India, since there is no specialized unit for toys in this territory. By taking into consideration the available resources, Toys and Dolls making industry, atleast, at medium scale level can be set up in different places of the Andaman and Nicobar Islands. The metal die cast toys-models of cars, engines, airplanes, electronic toys, handy battery operated video toys, stuffed toys, wooden toys, inflatable toys, squeeze toys, washable soft toys, bath toys etc. have excellent export prospects in the Bay Islands.

Available Resource

The Andaman and Nicobar Islands is rich in her resources. Besides the land resources, wood, rubber, plastic etc. are the prime raw materials for making of Toys and Dolls. As far as the wood is concerned, the forests cover about 86% of geographical area of the Island. Out of the 2,200 species of plants found in the forests about 200 species (10%) are endemic to the islands. It is estimated that about 3.63 lakhs cbm. of different varieties of wood as indicated below will be available annually on a sustained basis.

1.	Soft wood	0.75	lakhs	Cbm.
2.	Wood for Plywood	1.67	"	"
3.	Hard wood	1.21	"	"
	Total	3.63	"	"

The soil as well as agro-climatic conditions in these islands, particularly in the Nicobar group of islands, is suitable for the introduction of rubber plantation on a large scale. At present rubber plantation has been taken up in the South Andaman group and Katchal island in the Nicobar group of islands. So far 614 ha including 568 ha, raised by Rubber Board, have been covered. Latex, a product from the rubber plantation, is tapped. It is converted into rubber sheets and wholly exported to the mainland. The rubber production has been increasing fast every year which is shown in the Table No. 3.

Next to the wood and rubber, finance is an another input needed for any kind of activity. In the Andaman and Nicobar Islands, there are 7 banks - 6 commercial banks and 1 cooperative bank – with a total number of 37 branches. The Andaman and Nicobar State Cooperative Bank is the backbone of the cooperative credit facility. Besides, the bank credit, the District Industries Centre and Directorate of Industries, Port Blair also grant loans, incentives and subsidies under various schemes. The existence of interested entrepreneurs is another important factor to promote the proposed industry. In the Andaman and Nicobar Islands, the numbers of educated unemployed youths are quite big, and their number has been increasing. Under the Self Employment for Educated Unemployed Youths (SEEUY) scheme, the number of applications received is always more than the target number. This is very clear from the Table No. 4. This is also an evidence for the prospects for any industry in these islands. An interesting feature to be noted is that there is an increasing awareness of industries among the Schedule Tribes of the Andaman and Nicobar Islands.

Anticipated Problems

The Toys and Dolls Industry may have the following problems if started in the Bay islands.

1. Raw Material

For Toys and Dolls Industry, the wood and rubber are the prime raw materials. These are available in abundance in these islands. Very recently, the Chief Conservator of Forests (CCF) of these islands has issued a circular (vide letter No.F.10/G-1/7 dt. 14.3.86) that no new wood based industrial unit should be set up in these islands. The reason mentioned in the circular was that they do not have enough timber. At present, all the rubber production is exported to the mainland. There is no rubber processing industry in these islands atleast at small-scale level.

2. Technology

Another problem likely to affect the proposed industry is the absence of latest technology ad modernization. The reasons for this are the communication gap and transport problem. Once the industry is established, it will find difficult to introduce new technology by replacing the machineries due to the reasons mentioned above. Unless the proposed industry in this territory takes up modernization, it may find itself thrown out of business. It is advised that the entrepreneurs have to keep themselves abreast of developments in technology and to take up modernization.

3. Lack of Publicity

The lack of publicity is another problem in this territory. Neither the Andaman and Nicobar Administration nor the District Industries Centre / Directorate of Industries Port Blair does the publicity of the available resources, incentives, assistance, subsidies etc. Due to this problem, the infant entrepreneurs who need booster dose of the adequate information fail in the first stepping stage itself.

Suggestions

1. India's export of Toys and Dolls to the foreign countries has been about 200 lakhs every year. There is a good industrial climate for Toys and Dolls Industry in the Bay Islands. On the basis of the preceding discussions, it is suggested that two toy making units-one at Port Blair Region and the other at Rangat Region, six Doll making units-three at Port Blair Region, one each at Rangat, Mayabunder and Campbell Bay Regions – medium scale level, may be set up either by the Government Sector or by the private sector.
2. The Andaman and Nicobar Administration may immediately stop the export of latex rubber and rubber sheets and it may be made available as raw material for the proposed industry. The Administration has to establish a rubber processing unit atleast in medium scale level in the Bay Islands. The Administration may encourage the private sector to establish a processing unit in the territory itself. The Administration has to see that all the raw material production is supplied to the proposed units
3. Since it is an export-oriented industry, the Administration may extend all the possible helps to market the finished products of this proposed industry. Both the Administration and the entrepreneurs may share responsibilities. Advertisements are the booster doses whereas the delay on the part of the officers is the virus diseases, which will even, kill the entrepreneurs with family members. So the

Administration may take necessary steps to take decisions as quickly and early as possible without any Delay.

4. Electricity Department and Public Works Department may supply electricity without any cut and water with sufficient quantity, respectively.

Once the hindrances are removed and the Andaman and Nicobar Administration renders timely assistance without making delays to the interested entrepreneurs of the Toys and Dolls units, the Andaman and Nicobar Islands also can very well contribute its share to the mainland of India's exports of Toys and Dolls.

Table No. 1

Islands Divisions, Regions and Tehsils of A & N Islands

Islands	*Districts*	*Divisions*	*Regions*	*Tehsils*
Andaman & Nicobar Islands	1. Andaman	1. South Andaman	1. Port Blair 2. Ferrargunj	1. Port Blair 2. Ferrargunj
		2. North & Middle Andaman	3. Rangat 4. Mayabunder 5. Diglipur	3. Rangat 4. Mayabunder 5. Diglipur
	2. Nicobar	1. Carnicobar & Nancowry	1. Carnicobar 2. Nancowry 3. Campbell Bay	6. Carnicobar 7. Nancowry

Source: N. Rajavel, (1990).

Table No. 2

Toys and Dolls Requirement as per Age Group

Sl. No.	*Toys and Dolls*	*Average age when likely to start using Toys*	*Age upto which toys will remain in use*
1.	Rattles, pram beads, small	9 months	1 ½ years
	soft toys, soft blocks,	”	4 ”
	squeaking toys, baby shapes	”	2 ”
2.	Nursery rocker, washable	9 months	3 years
	soft toys, rag dolls	1 ½ years	3 ”
3.	Bath toys, baby walkers screwing toys	”	3 ”
4.	Wooden tram, easy couplings posting box, hammer bags	”	2 ½ ”

Sl. No.	*Toys and Dolls*	*Average age when likely to start using Toys*	*Age upto which toys will remain in use*
5.	Building beacons	"	3 "
6.	Large wooden animals (zoo or farm)	"	4 "
7.	Teddy bear and other soft toys	"	6 "
8.	Large wooden blocks, soft modeling material, wooden toys on casters to ride, floor toys, vehicles animals, ring figures, large lorry to load.	2-2 ½ years	5 "
9.	Dolls cot	"	9 "
10.	Climbing frame	"	12 "'
11.	Play bricks in bag (with related dimension)	2 ½ -3 years	10 "
12.	Small tricycles, train track (wooden railway)	"	7 "
13.	Tea set, first construction set, big wood pieces, farm building set, kitchen set, dolls, dolls pram, play town, miniature cars…….	3-4 years	8 "
14.	Sewing cards, clock with hands to move	4-5 years	6 "
15.	Construction toy picture lotto	" "	8 "
16.	Dolls, house dolls, house furniture dolls seals and weights, scooter, dressing up cloths, skipping rope, shanks and ladders ludo……	" "	10 "
17.	Mececano, Kaleidoscopes, Board	5-6 years	12 "
18.	Simple mechanical toys, simple electrical sets, battery operated toys…..	7-8 years	12 "

Table No. 3

Area and Production of Rubber in A & N Islands

Year	*Area (In Ha./)*	*Production (in Kg.)*
1981-82	598.84	88,800
1982-83	598.84	1,41,800
1983-84	598.84	2,46,600
1984-85	614.00	2,91,900
1985-86	614.00	4,61,000
1986-87	614.00	4,80,000
1987-88	614.00	4,94,000
1988-89	614.00	NA.
1989-90	615.00	4,90,000

Source: Basic Statistics of A&N Administration. NA – Not available

Table No. 4

Applications Received Cases Recommended and Amount Sanctioned Under S..E.EU.Y. Scheme

Year	*Target*	*Number of applications received*	*Number of cases recommended*	*Amount sanctioned (in Rs.)*
1983-84	100	256	112	14,97,000
1984-85	100	177	107	23,67,000
1985-86	100	218	119	24,56,000
1986-87	100	268	111a	16,10,000
1987-88	50	173	60b	18,77,000
1988-89	100	187	81c	14,72,000
1989-90	50	106	42	3,77,000

Source: DIC, Port Blair. Note: a - 6 STs; b - 1 ST; c - 4 ST.

11

MANUFACTURING INDUSTRY IN A&N ISLANDS – AN ANALYTICAL STUDY

Introduction

The maximum potential rate of growth of any country depends on the industrial development and the number of manufacturing units in the country. Manufacturing industry being the secondary sector to generate national income contributes significantly to the process of economic development. The rapid growth of industrial sector since Independence being one of the significant features of Indian economy, study of industrial units has acquired importance.

Andaman and Nicobar Islands is one of the important resourceful parts of the Indian Union. The manufacturing industry has an excellent scope for development and can play a vital role in the economic development of the islands. The District Industries Centre (DIC) and the Department of Industries (DI) of the study area call all the units registered as small scale units. No proper classification has been made so far and no study has been undertaken of the industrial sector in this area except the author's study on trade, commerce and industry. Hence an attempt has been made here to examine the manufacturing industry in this area in order to classify the manufacturing units on the basis of capital employed, raw material used and place of establishment; and, to identify the impediments and to offer suitable suggestions to overcome the problems.

Study Area

A&N Islands is situated in the Bay of Bengal, located between 6° and 14° NL and 92° and 94° EL. It is surrounded by Burma, Thailand, Malaysia and Indonesia, and is the most isolated part of the Indian Union. The Andaman group of island is separated from the Nicobar group by the boisterous 10 channel which is about 155 kms. Wide and 400 fathoms deep. This territory, comprising an area of 8,293 sq. kms is a group of picturesque islands. In all there are 319 islands; 258 islands in the Andaman group and 61 islands in the Nicobar group in the union territory of A&N islands. Of the total number, only 38 islands are inhabited. Port Blair, the capital of the territory, is connected with the mainland of India by both sea and air routes. The total population of this territory is 2,80,661: Andaman district consisting of 2,41,453 and Nicobar district 39,208. The territory is divided into two districts, three divisions and eight regions.* It is industrially backward. The economy of the A&N islands is comprised of agricultural sector, industrial sector and trading sector. The industrial sector can contribute a considerable share to the economy of A&N islands. The DIC and the DI have been calling all the units including units under tertiary sector as small-scale units. According to the DIC report to the A&N Administration, there are 869 small-scale units functioning in this territory.

Methodology

For the purpose of this study, the data were obtained from the DIC including the names and addresses of the units, year of establishment, products manufactured, capital employed on plant and machinery, business organisation, etc. From the main list, a separate list of manufacturing units has been prepared. On the basis of the location of the units, classification has been made as per the definition framed by the Government of India. Since the data could be collected only up to 1991, it was decided to classify the data as per the definitions prevailing in the year 1991 and as per the population data of the census year 1991. To highlight the problems of the units, about 60 units were visited and interviewed informally by the author. The identified problems and the data analysed are presented at the end of this paper.

Classification

From the list of industrial units, the total number of units identified and as manufacturing units for further classification was 339.

Capital Employed

Of the 339 units, as per the definition given by the Government of India, six (1.77%) are medium scale units, 18 (5.31%) small-scale units, 206 (60.77%) tiny units and 109 (32.15%) villages units (See table 1). Table 1 clearly reveals that there is no large-scale unit in the island; majority of the units area in the village and tiny sectors.

* Classified by the author in his doctoral dissertation.

Raw Material Used

This classification yielded the seven categories. They are: wood based (WBI), food based (FBI), sand and cement based (S&CBI), agro based (ABI), marine based (MBI), chemical based (CBI), and leather based (LBI).

The WBI consist of units which were manufacturing match splints, veneer, pencil slates, sawn timber, furniture, toys and dolls, etc. The FBI covers the units which were manufacturing bakery products, beverages vermicelli, chili sauce, papad, pickles, masala powder, vinegar etc. The MBI consists of only shell crafts units. The CBI included soaps, phenyl, candles, gas manufacturing units, etc. The ABI covers the units manufacturing oil, coir fibres, ropes, etc. The units manufacturing hollow block, bricks, posts, etc. are included under S & CBI. The LBI comprises units manufacturing shoes, chappals, suitcases, etc. (The classification of the units is shown in fig.1. The number of units under each category is given in table 2).

Ranking of industries based on the number of units is given in table3. the WBI with 187 units (55.16% of the total percent) ranks first followed by the FBI with 52 units (15.34%) placed in second rank. MBI consists of 37 units (10.92%) and ranks third, while the S & CBI with 36 units (10.62%) is in the fourth place. ABI ranks fifth with 14 units (4.13%) while CBI takes the sixth place with 9 units (2.65%). Lastly, the LBI is in the seventh place with only four units (1.18%). (The structure of the manufacturing industry in A&N Islands is shown in figure 2).

Region

As already stated the territory of A&N Islands is divided into two districts, three divisions and eight regions (Rajavel, 1990). Five of the eight regions – Port Blair, Ferrargunj, Rangat, Mayabunder and Diglipur – are situated in Andaman District and three regions – Car Nicobar, Nancowry and Campbell Bay – are in Nicobar District. The place where the actual manufacturing process is carried on has been taken as the basis for this classification. (The number of units region-wise and district-wise are shown in table 4).

Of the two districts, Andaman has a very large number of units (333 units representing 98.23% of the total) whereas Nicobar District has only six units (1.77%). From table 4, it becomes clear that among the regions of Andaman District, Port Blair has more number of units, (227 units comprising 68.17% of the total in Andaman District and 66.96% of the total number of units in the A&N Islands as a whole). Next to Port Blair, Rangat occupies the second place with 43 units (12.91%), followed by Ferrargunj region (8.11%), Diglipur region (6.01%) and Mayabunder region (4.81%). As far as the Nicobar District is concerned, there were no units in Nancowry region but four units (1.18% of the total units) were in Campbell Bay region and two units (0.59%) in Car Nicobar region.

Cross Analysis

A cross in-depth analysis has also been made region-wise and raw material-wise. The table clearly pictures that the units under WBI, FBI were found in almost all the regions except Car Nicobar and Nancowry regions. Of the 8 regions, Port Blair had 122 WBI units. This was 65.24% of the total units under WBI in the A&N Islands of which 30 units representing 57.69% of the total units under FBI, were situated in Port Blair region. Thirty units (81.08%) under MBI, 9 units (100%) under CBI, 6 units (42.86%) under ABI, 26 units (72.22%) under S & CBI, 4 units (100%) under LBI were situated in the Port Blair region. Absence of MBI units in Rangat region, Diglipur region and Nancowry region; WBI and FBI units in Car Nicobar region, and Nancowry region; ABI units in Mayabunder region, Nancowry region & Campbell region; A & CBI units in Mayabunder region and in all the regions of Carnicobar District; and CBI units and LBI units in all region except Port Blair region is an important notable fact. The main reason for the concentration of units in Port Blair region may be attributed to the availability of facilities, and the industrial awareness among the entrepreneurs of the city.

Another important cross analysis was made on the basis of raw material used and the capital employed. Table 6 shows the number of units classified raw material-wise and scale-wise. According to the table, majority of the units were under WBI. Except one unit out of the six medium scale units, all were wood based units. All the small scale sector units were wood based. Among the village and tiny units, out of 315 units 164 (52.06%) were wood based. The industrial development in the islands is still in the infant stage and not even in a developing stage, therefore, needs careful rethinking and revision of the whole system of industrialization of this territory.

Problems

The social, economic and geographical conditions of A&N Islands have restricted the emergence of creative industrial activities to a great extent. Consequently these islands, in spite of being very rich in natural resources, have remained industrially under-developed. In order to find out the problems facing the units in these islands, an informal study was conducted by the author, of about 60 units. The study revealed that the industrial units have faced numerous problems in course of promoting and constructing their units: extraordinary delay in getting registered, in getting power connection, water connection, and land conversion, in the preparation of feasibility report, in the selection of location, in procuring machinery etc. At the time of the study they were confronting a wide ranging operational problems related to adequate supply of power, raw material, transport, finance, marketing, delayed payment, inadequate working capital, labour shortage, provision for repairs, and communications. No doubt, the incentives, subsidies etc., provided by the central government and the local administration, and the different programmes offered by the commercial and cooperative banks are attractive but the industrial units in the Island find it difficult to enjoy these incentives and subsides due to various procedural complexities, intolerable delay on the part of the different organisations and indifferent attitude of the officials.

Summary of Findings and Suggestions

Given below is the summary of findings and some measures are suggested to solve the problems of the industrial units and for the overall development of industries in this territory.

1. Of the total units about 32 percent were village units, 61 percent tiny, 5 percent small scale and the rest of about 2 percent were medium scale units. There was no large-scale unit in this territory.

2. About 55 percent of the total units were wood based, 15 percent food based, 11 percent marine based, 11 percent sand and cement based, 4 percent agro based, 3 percent chemical based and only 1 percent was leather based. A large number (about 98%) of units were established in Andaman district and only 2 percent were in Nicobar district. Region wise, about 67 percent of the units were in Port Blair, 13 percent in Rangat, 8 percent in Ferrargunj, 6 percent in Diglipur, 5 percent in Mayabunder and about 1 percent each were in Campbell Bay and Car Nicobar.

3. Wood based and food based units were found in almost all the regions except in Car Nicobar and Nancowry. About 65 percent of the units under WBI, 100 percent of CBI units and LBI units, 72 percent of the units under S & CBI and about 43 percent of ABI units were situated in Port Blair region.

4. Absence of MBI units in Rangat, Diglipur and Nancowry regions, units under WBI and FBI in Car Nicobar and Nancowry regions, ABI units in Mayabunder, Nancowry and Campbell Bay regions, S & CBI

units in Mayabunder, Car Nicobar and Nancowry regions and the absence of units under CBI and LBI in all regions except Port Blair was a significant fact.

5. About 83 percent of medium scale units, 100 percent of small scale units and 52 percent of tiny ad village units were wood based.

6. Extraordinary delay in getting registration, power connection, water connection and land conversion were the problems faced by the units in the initial stage. Inadequate supply of power, water and raw materials, labour shortage, absence of market and market information, problems related to the provisions for repairs and communication were the difficulties faced at the operational stage.

7. The promoting agencies like DIC and DI should conduct an upto-date micro level study to keep trace of the registered and the unregistered units. They should organize contact programmes for the different industrialists so that, their common problems may be discussed and solved, the inter-industrial activities may be discussed, interactions between the industrialists themselves and between the officials and industrialists themselves and between the officials and industrialists may be made.

8. The facilities, subsidies, incentives, concessions, etc., available for the units and the type of assistance available at the DIC, DI, etc., are to be made known to the owners of the existing units and the prospective entrepreneurs. This may be accomplished through intensive advertisement and publicity. They can issue some video and audiocassettes on "How to start an industrial unit," "Hurdles in the development of industrial units," "Documents to be filed for registration." "Information about subsidies, incentives and other concessions," "Product development," "Market development", etc., to all the industrial units, or these cassettes may be screened at the time of the contact programme.

9. The unnecessary delay on the part of the government officers is to be totally avoided. Different officers involved in industrial development should meet at least once a month at a common place, preferably in the DIC premises. The industrialists, entrepreneurs, etc., may also be invited on the day. Their problems should be discussed and the proper approval and necessary sanctions must be granted on the same day so that the life killing delay will not occur.

10. The A&N Administration may procure the finished products of the local industrial units at fixed rates and those products may be exported to mainland. To facilitate this, the A&N Administration may establish sales counters at different places, preferably in cities and towns of the mainland.

11. Since rubber, plastic, coir, fish and marine, supari products, toys and dolls, garden furniture, household furniture have excellent export prospects the A&N Administration may call the investors for the setting up of 100 percent export oriented units in these product areas in the territory.

Conclusion

Once the impediments in the path of the industrial development in the A&N Islands are removed and an effective strategy is framed in the light of the above suggestions and adopted, the industrial activities will boost the economy of these islands.

Table 1

Number of units on the basis of capital employed (scale-wise)

Sl. No.	*Scale*	*No. of units*	*Percentage*
1.	Large Scale units	NIL	NIL
2.	Medium scale units	6	1.77
3.	Small scale units	18	5.31
4.	Tiny units	206	60.77
5.	Village units	109	31.15
	Total units	339	100.00

Table. 2

Number of units on the basis of raw material used (raw material-wise)

Sl. No.	*Raw material used*	*No. of units*	*Percentage*
1.	Wood based	187	55.16
2.	Food based	52	15.34
3.	Marine based	37	10.92
4.	Sand and cement based	36	10.62
5.	Agro based	14	4.13
6.	Chemical based	9	2.65
7.	Leather based	4	1.18
	Total units	339	100.00

Source : DIC Office, Port Blair (compiled).

Table 3

Ranking of industries based on the raw material used

S. No.	*Name of the industry*	*Rank*
1.	Wood based	I
2.	Food based	II
3.	Marine based	III
4.	Sand and cement based	IV
5.	Agro based	V
6.	Chemical based	VI
7.	Leather based	VII

Source : From Table 2.

Table 4

Number of units on the basis of region and district

Sl. No.	*Region / District / Islands*	*No. of units*	*Percentage*
1.	Port Blair R	227 (68.17)	66.96
2.	Ferrargunj R	27 (8.11)	7.96
3.	Rangat R	43 (12.91)	12.69
4.	Mayabunder R	16 (4.80)	4.72
5.	Diglipur R	20 (6.01)	5.90
	Andaman district	**333 (100.00)**	**98.23**
6.	Car Nicobar	2 (33.33)	0.59
7.	Nancowry R	--	--
8.	Campbell Bay R	4	1.18
	Nicobar District	**6 (100.00)**	**1.77**
	Andaman and Nicobar Islands	**339**	**100.00**

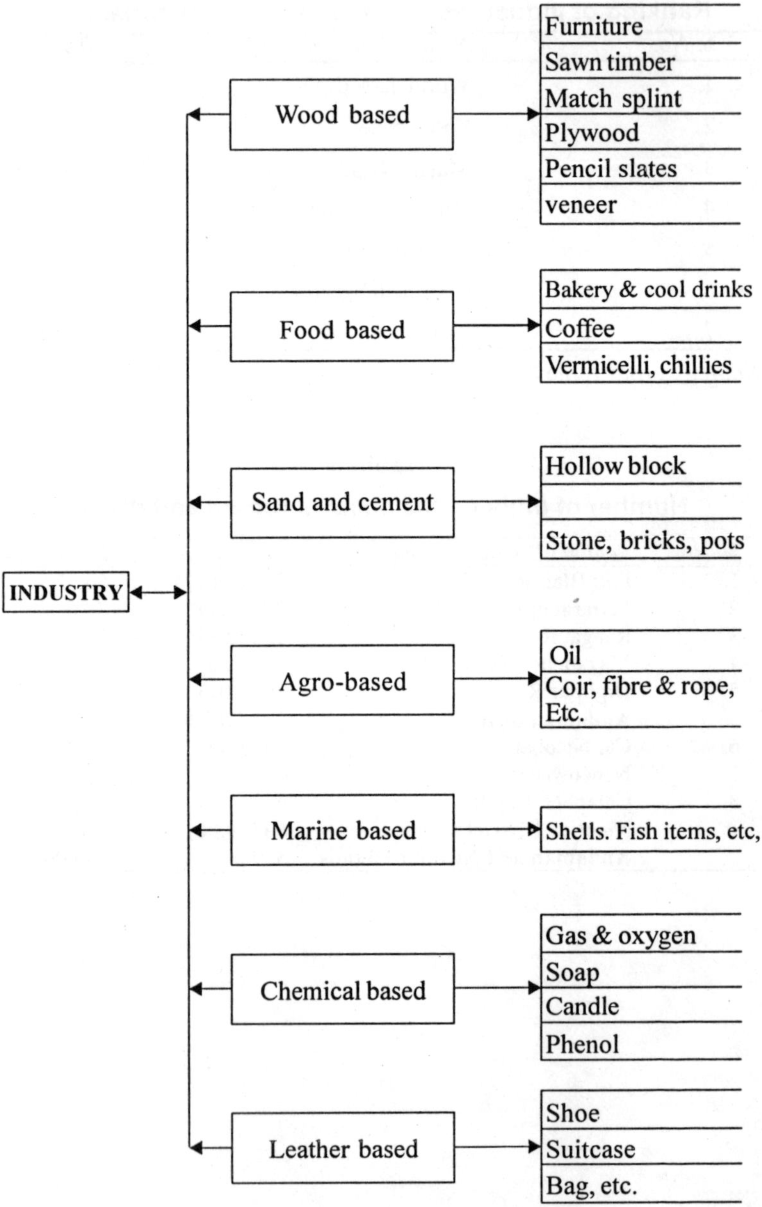
INDUSTRY
Wood based
Furniture
Sawn timber
Match splint
Plywood
Pencil slates
veneer
Food based
Bakery & cool drinks
Coffee
Vermicelli, chillies
Sand and cement
Hollow block
Stone, bricks, pots
Agro-based
Oil
Coir, fibre & rope, Etc.
Marine based
Shells. Fish items, etc,
Chemical based
Gas & oxygen
Soap
Candle
Phenol
Leather based
Shoe
Suitcase
Bag, etc.

12

Role of Banking Industry in the Economic Development of the Bay Islands

Introduction

Liberalization, Privatization, and Globalization are the recent tools and techniques adopted by many rapidly growing countries in the developing world. The major countries in the South Asia including India have been liberalizing their economies with a view to bring high growth rate in the forthcoming years. In India, particularly privatization is becoming made compulsory and felt compulsory to bring out reforms and to have an enhanced investment prospects in internal and external trade. Both liberalization as well as privatization in majority of the developing countries has proved success in developing their economy through the openings of financial activities like Banking, Mutual Funds, Pension Funds, Insurance and other commercial activities. These tools search the perspective possibilities of exploring the new ventures in industrial, commercial and trade activities from the available exploitable resources in the developing regions or the developing country. The present paper concentrates on the possibilities of financial market, investment opportunities in a fast developing union territory, Andaman & Nicobar Islands by taking the above mentioned tools and techniques of development and economic reforms as key points.

Presently the different sectors of the economy of A & N islands get the financial assistance both from the Institutions and Non-Institutions. Institutional finance is a financial assistance given by the established institutions like commercial banks, cooperative banks, government departments, insurance companies etc.. Non institutional finance is the financial assistance given by the professional money lenders, traders, commission agents, relatives, friends, chit fund organisations etc.

Bay Islands Since Independence

Bay islands i.e the Andaman and Nicobar Islands, by virtue of its strategic geographical location in the Bay of Bengal and rich Natural Resources, attracts and receives great attention. The Bay Islands, as it is also known, constitute the remotest region of our country. The inky, blue waters of the Bay of Bengal and the Andaman Sea, once coined as KALAPANI (the Black water) indicating the dreaded transportation, punishment of the British Government of India and the overwhelming grandeur of vast, cloud ridden skies make them a domain of unsullied nature. "KALAPANI" is all that many have heard of a term that for centuries conjured up the dark vision of forbidden land surrounded by vast sheets of deep water, unapproachable and hostile. The inhabitants of these islands are scattered far flung and wide over a distance of 720 Kms. Some of them are found established well in a few towns and innumerable small villages. But due to the location of these small villages, inhabitants are cut-off from civilization and from the source of supply of essential commodities .The towns and small villages have started flourishing only recently, because of the horbour facilities that have been provided in these islands and slow progress of shipping and other transport facilities. Andaman and Nicobar islands is a green paradise which stretches its long arm of welcome to the mainland across the sea, an outpost pulsating some pioneering activities.

The population of Andaman & Nicobar Islands when we gained Independence was just 30,000 of which the tribal population was about 12,000. Since Independence, the population started increasing, people from the mainland started finding these islands suitable for living, Administration also invited people from mainland for the settlement, Jobs were vacant in every field, possibilities of setting the industrial units have become visible, academicians, anthropologists, economists, researchers identified the resources etc., These great changes have now induced the social scientists, anthropologists to be engaged in the study of the social and economic change.

A & N Islands, situated in the Bay of Bengal are surrounded by Burma, Thailand, Malaysia and Indonesia. The islands constitute the most isolated part of Indian Union, stretching in North South direction, separated from the Mainland of India vast stretches of sea. The Andaman groups of islands are separated from Nicobar group of islands by 10o channel. This territory, comprising an area of 8293 square kilometers, is a group of picturesque islands. Port Blair, the capital of these Bay Islands is connected with the Mainland by both sea and air routes. The population of A & N Islands is 2, 80,661 as per the census year 1991 and 3,56,265 as per the census year 2001. The seat of Administration is situated in Port Blair City.

Ingredients of the Economy

Only from the recent past, these Islands witness some growth, which can be counted for economic development. Number of industrial units, trade units, commercial units, travel units started increasing by showing a growing trend at a lower rate. The Chamber of Commerce & Industry Associations of Small-Scale Units and trade associations have been contributing their possible efforts to the growth of these islands. But all such valuable efforts couldn't bring the expected result due to some unsolvable problems at our end which are pushing down the economy of the A & N Islands to the infant stage status. However, the Govt. of India, if desired can solve such unsolvable problems.

Each and every aspects and transactions is no doubt, responsible for the economic development of this territory. Of all, the major and main ingredients are Agriculture, Trade, Commerce, Industry and Tourism. Agriculture is the backbone of our Indian Economic System since it is the supplier of food. Industry plays an important role by providing employment opportunity, meeting consumer needs, help in resource utilization, accelerating economic growth, mobilizing manpower, promoting self-employment. As far as the trade is concerned, the domination of internal import trade is the more than the internal export trade. But sill the trade plays a very vital role by mobilizing and transferring the goods and services from the different parts of the mainland to these islands and from one island to another island. In a research work on Problems and Prospects of trade, Commerce and Industry in A & N Islands by the author of this article, Trade Activity is named as " LIFE GIVING ASPECT" to the people of A & N islands. Commerce i.e. transports banking, storage, insurance and advertisement contributes its share to some extend. Of all the banking plays an important role in the development of all economic activities. Tourism, a smokeless industry is also one of the major ingredients of the economy. Though it is in infant stage it stretches its arms by inviting a large number of visitors and investors. The roles of Trade, Commerce, Industry and Tourism in the economic development of A & N Islands are the excellent and are opened for healthy Seminar and the concerned departments are to be motivated for the organization of such Seminars for the further development.

Prospects

Once A & N Islands was coined as "KALAPANI" a black water. But it is no more Kalapani now. No doubts, this territory gains a lot of developments in every field. But the rate of growth is very low. What NOT available in these islands? It has everything here. Why should it depend upon Mainland for everything? One can make the Mainland to depend upon these islands. Now what is going here is that all goods are sent at raw level to the mainland and the finished goods are purchased from there. The betelnut/arecaunut (supari) is sent to mainland at raw level but the finished products of the arecaunut line like sugandh supari, scented supari, seeval supari, pan parag etc are purchased. In the same manner the coconuts are sent but the coconut oil and oil cake are purchased from the mainland and like this many products at its raw level are sent to mainland which is against the principles of comparative advantages. There are no toys and dolls industry in these islands at small-scale level, which has excellent market potentiality both in mainland and abroad. Casuarinas plantation, Mango plantation, Eucalyptus plantation, Coconut plantation, Cashew plantation, and Arecaunut plantation show encouraging results. All these cash crop plantations will certainly increase the income of territory in long run by promoting number of small- scale units. This territory has historical resources for tourism industry. By its multiplier effect, the tourism industry helps in increasing the economic development. So, a number of small scale units on new areas like inter-island transport, inter-island communication service, mainland-island air service, power, coconut oil, arecaunut based seeval and supari, marine goods like fish, prawn, shells, sea cucumber, and other available resources. Hence, this territory has excellent potentiality and prospects for all the economic activities.

Banking – Responsible for Change

Finance is the life blood of each and every economic activity. It brings the changes in the socio economic and even cultural surface. Without finance nothing is possible in the present scenario. It plays a vital role in the functions of the factors responsible for the socio economic changes. There are many factors responsible for Socio-economic changes of Andaman & Nicobar Islands. Such factors are identified. They are Demographic Factor, Technological Factor, Cultural Factor, Revolution Factor, War Factor, Legislation Factor, Planning Factor, Education Factor, Trade Factor, Commerce Factor, Industrial Factor, and Tourism Factor. Actually, the changes are the result of the effective role of one or more of these factors on the Socio-economic surface of the particular region or country or area. Actually finance is the base for all factors and that plays a very vital role in each and every field.

Finance – The Present Scenario

The present scenario of the finance in these islands is very interesting to study and note. Though the area is small, here the financial transactions are going proportionately not less than the transactions of the mainland. Rate of interest is also very interesting. The Finance Sector of the Andaman and Nicobar Islands is divided into two Organised Sector and Un-Organised Sector.

Organised Sector

Organised Sector consists of 03 types of intuitions namely Commercial Banks, Cooperative Banks and NABARD. The Commercial Banks includes State Bank of India, Indian Bank, Canara Bank, Indian Overseas Bank, Punjab National Bank, UCO Bank. Allahabad Bank, United Bank, and Vijaya Bank. The Andaman and Nicobar Islands State Cooperative Bank consists of 31 branches. The Growth of Organised sector is shown in the table.

Table 1

Growth of Organised Financial Institutions (in Nos.)

Sl. No.	*Year*	*No. of Branches*	*Rate in %*
01	1970	04	--
02	1975	11	175.0
03	1980	24	118.2
04	1985	32	33.3
05	1990	47	46.9
06	1995	56	19.2
07	2000	64	14.3

Source: Compiled from the Basic Statistics.

Un-Organised Sector

As far as the Un-Organised Sector is concerned, financial assistance given by the professional money lenders, traders, commission agents, relatives, friends, chit fund organisations etc. The data on traders, relatives and friends who lend money to others could not be collected. However, the data on the moneylenders, commission agents, chit fund organisations have been collected personally by meeting the aged people of different regions. The surprising news is that there is one type of money lending named "Kenthu Vatti". Kenthu Vatti means giving money for very short period at heavy rate of interest. Say for example, if a man gets money Rs. 1000 on Kenthu Vatti today by 1700 Hrs. tomorrow he has return the money before 1700 Hrs. along with the interest of Rs. 250 – Rs. 500 depending upon the Kenthu Vatti Moneylender and upon the urgency and position of the money taker. There are incidents that interest alone will become equal to the principal amount for a day. Who are doing this Kenthu Vatti business ? is another question. Educateds particularly in the Teaching line are showing serious importance and interest in doing this business. The following table shows the growth of this unorganized sector in terms of the persons involved in the money lending business.

Table 2

Growth of Un-Organised Sector – Persons (in Nos.)

S. No.	*Year*	*No. of Persons*	*Rate in %*
01	1970	86	–
02	1975	121	40.7
03	1980	182	50.4
04	1985	292	60.4
05	1990	467	59.9
06	1995	790	69.2
07	2000	1460	84.8

Source: Personal Collection – 2000.

Banking and Socio-Economic Changes

As is already told that the banking industry is the base for only hope of the economic growth of these islands. Banking, in terms of number of units has recorded a marvelous and significant growth Shortage of capital, shortage of entrepreneur, shortages of entrepreneurial ability, shortage of skills, shortage of technical know- how, inadequacies of transport, inadequate credit system were the situation of Andaman & Nicobar Islands. However, for the purpose of colonization, the people were brought form mainland and even they were given free lands and other facilities for other developmental purpose. Inefficient and corrupt officers were the major political factor, which threatened the economic development of Andaman & Nicobar Islands. But now, the whole scenario started changing. Socio-economic changes have started their visibilities in the following areas due to the growth of banking industry in Andaman & Nicobar Islands.

1. Number of educational institutions
2. Caste system
3. Cultural system
4. Status of women
5. Upliftment of tribals
6. Number of industrial units
7. Number of commercial units
8. Employment
9. Per capita income
10. Small savings
11. Entertainment
12. Capital mobilization - many entrepreneurs have started coming to Andaman & Nicobar Islands to begin new ventures.

Though there are many numbers of elements in the Socio economic system of our Bay islands, the following elements are taken for this present paper to examine the changes due to tourism. Data has been collected and with the help of statistical tool called correlation analysis, the relationship has been examined.

1. Education
2. Savings
3. Trade & Commerce
4. Industries and
5. Employment

Banking and Education

Education plays a very vital role in the process of human resource development. Number of educational institutions namely schools, colleges, and institutions etc. has been increasing significantly. The banking industry has a close positive correlation with the increase in number of educational institutions. What I want to say is that the education is one of the aspect of the social system and that too very important organ of the social system. For the increase of educational institutions, banking growth is not the only the reason but that is also one of the reasons/ causes. But the growth of banking industry has been compelling the administration to go for a separate courses on banking. The following table shows the growth educational institutions due to the growth of banking.

Table 3
Education & Banking

Sl. No.	Year	No. of Branches	Change	Edu.Inst. In Nos	Change
01	1970	04	–	104	–
02	1975	11	+ ve	217	+ ve
03	1980	24	+ ve	243	+ ve
04	1985	32	+ ve	284	+ ve
05	1990	47	+ ve	321	+ ve
06	1995	56	+ ve	341	+ ve
07	2000	64	+ ve	361	+ ve

Source: Compiled from the Basic Statistics, Annual Reports of A & N Administration, Rajavel, 1990.

Banking and Savings

Savings is another important element of the social system. Savings is one of the factors determining the economic growth also. When other things remain constant, one can say that when income increases, the savings will also increase. There a lot of ways in which the income can be increased. Tourism is also one of the source of income of the people of Andaman & Nicobar Islands. Number of tourist travel agencies and their increase, increase in applications for the tourist and travel agency, increase in hotels and restaurants are the evidence for the tourism activity as one of the source of income. All such ingredients of the tourism is the result of increase in banks in Andaman and Nicobar Islands. They provided financial support and assistance to such units. These resulted in the multiplier effect of income generation which pushes the savings up. The statistical analysis shows the growth of banks and the growth savings have positive correlation. The following table shows the growth of savings due to growth of banks.

Table. 4
Banking and Savings

S.No.	Year	No. of Branches	Change	Savings In Lakhs	Change
01	1970	04	--	28	--
02	1975	11	+ve	72	+ve
03	1980	24	+ve	110	+ve
04	1985	32	+ve	183	+ve

S.No.	Year	No. of Branches	Change	Savings In Lakhs	Change
05	1990	47	+ve	422	+ve
06	1995	56	+ve	735	+ve
07	2000	64	+ve	1337	+ve

Source: Compiled from the Basic Statistics, Annual Reports of A & N Administration, Rajavel, 1990.

Banking and Trade and Commerce

Trade and commerce are the elements of economics and are the life giving aspects of these islands. If these elements favourably record the growth, then one can see the economic developments. Other wise the problems will be the result. The growth of trade and commerce has directly related with the growth of financial institutions. It may not be true in the mainland but in these islands, it is true at least to the extent of 70% though not 100%. Trade units, commercial establishments like different offices, restaurants, theaters etc are coming up based upon the needs and urges. Such needs and urges are met only by increasing banking industry. Again here also, the statistical analysis has recorded a positive correlation between the tourists arrival and number of trade and commercial units in Andaman & Nicobar Islands. The following table shows the growth of banks and trade units.

Table 5

Banking and Trade and Commerce

Sl. No.	*Year*	*No. of Branches*	*Change*	*Shops In Nos*	*Change*
01	1970	04	–	379	–
02	1975	11	+ve	515	+ve
03	1980	24	+ve	813	+ve
04	1985	32	+ve	868	+ve
05	1990	47	+ve	965	+ve
06	1995	56	+ve	1,071	+ve
07	2000	64	+ve	1,220	+ve

Source: Compiled from the Basic Statistics, Annual Reports of A & N Administration, Rajavel, 1990.

Banking and Industries

Industries are the major determinant and the scale to measure the economic development of any region and so the case of Andaman &

Nicobar Islands also. The more number of inflow of tourists and their increasing purchase and buying habits encourage the industrial entrepreneurs to set up many units. Increase in number of units means decrease in problems of the Socio- economic System because such increase will create and increase the employment opportunities, identification of new ventures, capital mobilization, labour mobilization, one unit will create opportunity for the next and new unit etc. This will have multiplier effect in the Socio-economic system. The increasing number of banks has a positive correlation with the increase in number of industrial units. The following table shows the increase in number of banks and industrial units.

Table 6

Banking and Industries

Sl. No.	*Year*	*No. of Branches*	*Change*	*Industrial Units In Nos.*	*Change*
01	1970	04	--	46	--
02	1975	11	+ve	97	+ve
03	1980	24	+ve	156	+ve
04	1985	32	+ve	471	+ve
05	1990	47	+ve	869	+ve
06	1995	56	+ve	1180	+ve
07	2000	64	+ve	1374	+ve

Source: Compiled from the Basic Statistics, Annual Reports of A & N Administration, Rajavel, 1990.

Banking and Employment

This is another important economic as well as social factor which will determine the quality of the society, quality of the economy and the Socio-Economic Growth of any region and country and so the case of Andaman & Nicobar Islands also. For any economy, the major problem is the unemployment problem, which is the chronicle reason for all such anti-national, causes activities. But the Banking Industry reduces that burden considerably through its effective role in the Socio-economic system of Andaman & Nicobar Islands. As is already pointed out that the educational institutions, industrial units, etc. have been increasing due to the increasing economic activity of the Banking Industry. As a result the employment in the private trade and commercial establishments besides the government employment has also shown a positive growth with positive correlation with the increase in number of tourists into these islands. The following tables shows the increase in banks and increase in employment.

Table 7

Banking and Employment

Sl. No.	*Year*	*No. of Branches*	*Change*	*Employment In Nos.*	*Change*
01	1970	04	--	819	--
02	1975	11	+ ve	1178	+ ve
03	1980	24	+ ve	1985	+ ve
04	1985	32	+ ve	2410	+ ve
05	1990	47	+ ve	2569	+ ve
06	1995	56	+ ve	3985	+ ve
07	2000	64	+ ve	5248	+ ve

Source: Compiled from the Basic Statistics, Annual Reports of A & N Administration, Rajavel, 1990.

Correlation Analysis

To find out the co-relations between the changes in number of branches in the organised finance sector i.e increase in number of branches and the changes in the economy, correlation analysis is being undertaken. The number of branches in these islands has been correlated with the different aspects of the economy namely, Educational Institutions, Savings, Shops i.e. Commercial Establishments, Industrial units and the Employment generated to test the influence of the Banking Industry on the Economy of the Andaman and Nicobar Islands. Surprisingly it gives a positive coefficient of correlation at high value. The values of the coefficient of correlation are given below.

Table 8

Influence of Banking Industry on the Economy

Sl. No.	*Correlation between Banking and*	*Coefficient Value*
1	Educational Institutions	0.944628412
2	Small Savings	0.890050811
3	Commercial Establishments	0.977327481
4	Industrial Units	0.975950499
5	Employment Generated	0.954445496

Source: Calculated by the Author- 2003.

Prospects for Financial Market

1. A & N Islands has potential resources. Majority of the resources are unexploited and under exploited. May be due to the government policy, bureaucratism, Politics, lack of knowledge etc., the economic development of these islands, in spite of plannable, industrial, and potential resources, could not and do not record a markable growth rate. Absence of clear- cut industrial policy and proper guidelines, absence of effective orientations to the existing and intending investors and the entrepreneurs. A & N Islands is rich in her forest resources, marine resources, plantations resources, human resources and the potential natural beauty resources. Out of the total geographical area of about 8249 sq. km., it is still reported that 86% is under forest cover. About 41000 hectares of land are being used for the cultivating various crops namely Paddy, Coconut tree, Arecaunut, Fruits, Spices, Rubber, Red Oil Palm etc. It also reported that experiment trial and the pilot projects on Coffee, Clove, Nutmeg, and Cinnamon and Pepper have shown encouraging and profitable results. Banking Sector can have its more scope and expand its area, if proper planning and strategy is made and implemented.

2. Forests of A & N Islands are unique in character and possess enormous biological diversity. Out of 15000 flowering plants in India, 2200 spices are found in these island and among them 200 spices (10%) are endemic to these islands, about 1300 spices are not found in the main land of the country. Besides, these islands have high-valuable and high commercial valued medicinal plants and products like Amber, Hawabill are also available plenty in this territory. This territory, with its 1960 kms of coastline, has clearly a vast, owned valuable and potential fishery resources. Commercial fishes like Tuna, Seer, Marline and Saw Fish and Sharks etc. are found in abundance in these waters. It is supported by the evidences of the apprehension of foreign vessels, which came into these islands for fishing. Besides fish, Turtles, Sea Water Crabs and summer Crabs, Beach-de-mer (Sea Cucumber), Corals, Prawns etc are some of the high commercial valued marine wealth. In Andaman and Nicobar Islands till date, effective Industrial Policy is not made. With the available resources mentioned above, if a proper policy is drafted by having the open discussions with the Banking Industry, no doubt, the above mentioned resources will have meaning in the developmental process in the economy of the Andaman and Nicobar Islands.

3. These islands have a unique tropical Eco-system within expected wide range of genetic diversity and wild germ plasm as natural beauty. The biotic conditions and the climate of these islands are essentially congenial for high productivity. The rich Mangrove Eco- system, different species of Flora and Fauna, under water coral life, sandy beaches and wonderful creeks and unpolluted environment are the potential resources to attract the international and the domestic tourists. Moreover, one of these islands is situated nearby to the international maritime route. In Andaman and Nicobar Islands till date, no tourism policy is made. With the available tourism resources mentioned above, if a proper policy is drafted by having the open discussions with the Banking Industry, no doubt, the above mentioned resources will increase the economic development of the Andaman and Nicobar Islands.

4. As is already mentioned that the government of India is in the favour of liberalization and privatization, the views of the same may be implemented with full scope and hope, in this territory by taking the level of exploitable resources available in this territory. Required number of commercial banks is functioning in this territory. The government of India and the local government may encourage the setting up of large- scale industries through liberalization by inviting the private sectors. Who in turn will work out their functions with the growing Banking Sector.

5. At present the power is produced by the government sector with a number of problems of self and to the public due to many reasons. The power sector may be privatized and the required funds and the capitals are to be mobilized either locally or from the mainland. Communication is another area, which require immediate attention with the requirements of capitals. The government of India has to invite the private sector to set up an Inter Island. Communication unit including postal, telegraphs, telecommunication, information technologies and the related services.

6. Tourism, a smokeless industry has a high potential and prospects in the territory. Individual islands may be allotted to private sectors on contract basis without distributing the security affairs to set up and establish the tourism aspects with a view to attract costly tourists. The quickest mode of transport is Air Transport but at present the people of A & N Islands, the tourists both domestic as well as foreign and the government officials are going to Inter Islands by boat only.

The private sector may be encouraged to establish helicopter service and fast going ferry/boat service. Like wise, the education and higher education may be thought of for privatization.

7. The Andaman & Nicobar Administration may construct single room accommodation at very cheaper rate in the important places of interest of A & N islands. The administration may think for the floating accommodations. For that purpose, the Private Sectors may be called and encouraged. The hotels and restaurants who face the off-season problems may adopt and announce the multiple concession schemes like discount during off-season, meals on no profit no loss basis, more % of concession if they stay for more period, family tourist concession etc. The Andaman & Nicobar Administration may introduce Island Air Service. A detailed scheme is given in tourism book Tourism in Andaman & Nicobar Islands written by the author about the method of operation. Accommodation facilities for the tourists who wish to come to and go from Andaman & Nicobar Islands may be constructed near the horbour and the airport. Cable cars, Rope ways, Bus Terminus for the private buses, are to be constructed in the Port Blair.

Suggestions

To increase the role of the banking sector in the economy of the green resourceful paradise Andaman and Nicobar Islands, the following measures are suggested. The banking sector and its function in the mainland can not be equalized to these islands. One may not rather should not talk about the functions by equalizing the island and the mainland. There are a lot of reasons for such differences.

1. First, the awareness about the banking is to be brought in among the rural islands. Because, majority of the rural population have very less knowledge about the banking industry. They see, feel, and look in a surprising way when we talk about the banking industry. If one goes on talk about the rules and regulations, why should we go and tell and bring the awareness among the population particularly the rural population, then there will not be any solution for any problem.

2. Secondly, even some of the educated people have less knowledge about the banking transactions, procedures, available facilities, services provided by the banking industry, documents to be submitted to avail a loan or any facility etc., They feel highly embarrassed if they go to the banks. Because what we talk is entirely different from what we act in practice. So, the banking industry must come forward to make awareness in the minds of all both living in

urban and rural by leaving the arguments regarding why should we give such awareness etc.

3. The un-organised sector of the Moneylenders, Kenthu Vatti agents, Commission agents, Chit funds etc., are to be brought in a organised sector. They are to be called and open discussion is to be made with them regarding what they want to come in the organised sector. They are to be told to register themselves and the rate of interest to be charged by them is to be determined in a combined way of dialogues.

4. The above-unorganized sector people are to be identified and they are to be brought in the income tax brackets. They may be allowed to do their business according to their own ways but with the knowledge of the government. Government servants who are doing and actively involved either directly and indirectly may be instructed to submit the information and facts to the government.

5. Now the Banking Sector has the weekly holiday on every Sunday. If it is the case, the employees who are having the weekly holiday on Sunday find it very difficult to go and complete the banking transactions. Sometimes it takes months together to do a small work in the bank. This problem is more acute to the sincere, dedicated and duty bound employees. So it is suggested that the Banking Industry may have their weekly holiday in any day other than Sunday.

6. The banking sector gives loan to the employees by adopting number of formalities. I am not telling every formality is unnecessary. But their activities contain many unnecessary formalities. That may be avoided without any problem to the industry. Some formalities are kept due to the ignorance of the policy makers. So unnecessary formalities may be avoided.

7. One of the formalities while availing loan is that the loanee officer/ employee has to submit a letter from the Drawing and Disbursing Officer (DDO) of the institution where the employee is working. But generally, the DDOs are not giving the certificate/letter. They can not issue such certificates or letters to anyone . As a result, the employee finds it very difficult to avail the loan facility from the bank. Here both the bank as well as the employees face problems and in particular the bank loses the interest income. Generally, the managers do not take this matter seriously. It is a matter of personal talk with the DDO and the controlling officer of the DDO of the offices. If possible, it is suggested that the managers may call a meeting with the controlling officers and DDOs and discuss the matter in the meeting and can get concurrence.

8. The top level management of the Banking Sector must take up the matter at higher level in such a way every DDO must be provided with a manual regarding this issue and they are to be authorised to issue such forms by their controlling officers and the necessary powers are to be delegated to the DDOs.
9. It is suggested that the Banking sector may further extend business hours atleast for another one hour in the evening with the restrictions of the deposit, withdrawal and Demand Drafts on Savings Banks Accounts. Banks are the only institutions living totally on the deposit holders money. So the banks must instruct the employees of the banks to move very politely with the deposit holders. Some of the employees of the banks do pose too much as if they are giving money from their pocket when a deposit holder goes for the withdrawal of his own money. The deposit holders are made ashamed and they feel to go out of the bank and they leave bank without doing any transactions. Here every one is not blamed there are excellent employees in the banking sector who gives and takes care of the deposit holders.

Conclusion

The Banking Sector has brought marvelous changes in the education, employment, industrial units, trade & commerce and savings. It is the evidence from the correlation analysis that there is close correlation between the above areas and sector and the Banking Industry. Capitals are to be mobilized to create a comparative advantage. So by having a thorough study, a suitable and practical strategy is to be framed and the same may be carefully implemented. Possibilities and prospects for the establishment of different type of units are more in these islands. The local administration should invite the private sector ventures to invest in the prospective identified units/areas by realizing the importance, benefits of the new approach of economic reform namely Liberalization, Privatization and Globalization. The capital market will definitely bring a considerable and markable growth in the economy of these green islands. The capital mobilization and the market for capitals can be emerged only if the ample number of industries, at small, medium and large-scale with the benefits of liberalization and privatization, are established in this territory and a large number of areas are allocated to the private sector in this territory. Once, the strategy is formulated in the light of the above suggestions, I hope that th. Banking Industry will definitely increase the economic growth of this green paradise on the blue surface.

13

Power and Business Concerns in the Bay Islands

Abstract

A & N Islands is rich in resources of which only a very few have been exploited. The business activities have excellent prospects in these islands. But for the want of infrastructural facilities particularly power which plays a vital role in the development of business concerns, the economy of the Bay Islands could not be developed. The consequences of power problem on business concerns in A & N Islands are dealt in the present paper. Suggestions to remove the constraints faced by the business concerns due to power shortage are derived after careful analysis based on the data collected through the questionnaires.

Introduction

After penal settlement, in A & N Islands, the local inhabitants as well as the migrants are trying to establish wood based, marine based industries and some of them are running well. Apart from the industrial units, business concerns mushroomed in this union territory to provide the basic needs of the population. Both industrial units and trade concerns in this territory depend greatly on the mainland (India) for all the commodities. Industrial units, trade concerns and other commercial enterprises for their production and sales greatly depend on power. The main source of power is electricity generated by diesel generators. As there is no other source of power supply, hence there is always a shortage of power affecting the industrial production and business economy. Keeping in view of power as the key point, a study was conducted to analyse the consequences of power shortage on business concerns as no such study was conducted earlier.

Study Area

A & N Islands consisting of 572 islands, rocks and hillocks, lie in the Bay of Bengal, is about 1200 kms. away from Madras and Calcutta, have good potential of natural resources and offer better prospects for business activities inhabited in 35 islands. The details of these islands are described somewhere else by the author (Rajavel 1992).

Methodology

To collect the primary data concerned with the nature and types of power problems and its consequences, a semi-structured questionnaire was prepared and administered on selected business units through sampling technique. Business concerns include trade units and industrial units. It was decided to select 10% of the units in each region. In order to cover all the islands in each region and to have proper representation, it was decided to select 1 or 2 units from each island though the number of units exceeds 10%. In all 160 units were selected for sample but the total number of effective sample units was only 129 units. Particulars of sample units are given in Table 1. The author had visited many units to verify the problems. The collected data were analysed and are presented.

Table 1

Particulars of Sample Units

Sl. No.	*Particulars*	*Number of Units under*		*Total*
		Trade	*Industry*	
1.	Number of selected units	90	70	160
2.	Questionnaire mailed	90	70	160
3.	Units did not reply	03	07	10
4.	Remaining	87	63	150
5.	Units using manpower as motive power	–	21	21
6.	Number of effective sample units	87	42	129

Islands On March, A & N Administration, Port Blair, March 24.

Results and Discussion

The Table 2 shows the number of business units face power problem. The table also reveals that out of 129 units, 99 units representing 76.7 % face power problems while only 23.3% do not face such problem. When compared the industrial units with the trade units, the industrial units have more problems, that is, about 85% of the industrial units face the problem. 64 trade units representing 73.6% of the total sample trade units face the power problem. The further analysis is related to the nature (consequences) of the problem due to the inadequate power supply. The consequences are analysed and discussed in three categories namely Category I, II, and III.

Table 2

Power Problems and Business Concerns

Sl. No.	*Business Concerns*	*FP*	*NFP*	*Total*
1.	Industrial Units	35 (83.3)	7 (16.7)	42 (100.0)
		(35.4)	(23.3)	(32.6)
2.	Trade Units	64 (73.6)	23 (26.4)	87 (100.0)
		(64.6)	(76.7)	(67.4)
3.	Total	99 (76.7)	30 (23.3)	129 (100.0)
		(100.0)	(100.0)	(100.0)

Source: Primary Data 1992 Note: FP- Facing Problem NFP- Non Facing Problem.

Category I

This includes the problems of low capacity utilisation, high cost of production and loss of man-days faced by the units particularly industrial units due to inadequate power supply. The problem ultimately affects the overall performance of a unit or units. This problem has its reflections in the performance, which gives an idea of the magnitude of the problem. So the author has assumed that capacity utilisation of a unit gives a true and fair view of the performance, i.e, unutilized capacity of any unit is an indeed of its problem. Table 3 gives the data relating to the number of the units facing low capacity utilisation (average annual unutilized capacity). Table 4 gives data relating to the number of units facing the problem under category I for all 42 units under survey.

Table 3

Distribution of Average Unutilized Capacity

Sl. No.	*Unutilized Capacity*	*Number of Units*	*Percentage*
1.	Below 25%	02	5.7
2.	25% - 50%	11	31.4

3.	50% - 75%	16	45.7
4.	75% - 100%	06	17.2
	Total	35	100.0

Source: Primary Data 1992.

As per the Table 3 only 2 units (5.7%) had unutilized capacity to the extent of less than 25%. On the other extreme 6 units (17.2%) ah unutilized capacity of 75% and above. The unutilized capacity of 45.7% of the units is ranging between 50% - 75% and for about one third (31.4%) of the units; it is 25% - 50%. As per table 4, 34 units representing 97.1% of the units facing power problem reported that their cost of productions heavily increasing and 25 units representing 71.4% of the units facing power problem said that they face the problems of loss of man- days due to the inadequate power supply.

Table 4

Number of Units Facing Problems under Category I

Sl. No.	*Nature of Problem*	*Number of Units (out of 35)*	*Percentage*
1.	Low capacity Utilisation	33	94.3
2.	High cost of Production	34	97.1
3.	Loss of Man days	25	71.4

Source: Primary Data 1992.

Category II

This category includes problems faced both by the industrial and trade units. The problems are attractions of customers by the competitors, customers, dissatisfaction, loss of business and increase in overhead expenses. Customer creation is of the major objectives of every prudent business unit. When customers are eagerly coming to the units, if the power goes off means, the whole business opportunity is going out. Some business units are fully equipped with mini generators with a help of which they attract not only the customers but also the customers of the other units. While expressing their difficulties, all the business units facing such difficulties mentioned that such power cuts are cutting their throats. Table 5 shows the number of units facing the problems under the category.

As per the Table 5, of the 99 units facing the power problem 76 units representing 76.8% have expressed that their competitors due to this power problem attract their customers. Seventy-six units include 54 (83.4%) trade units and 22 (62.9%) industrial units. Next to this problem, customer dissatisfaction is another painful problem to the business units. Generally, a satisfied customer is a best advertiser and on the other hand a dissatisfied customer may go against the business unit. To a great surprise, out of 99 units under sample facing power problem, 94 units representing 95% informed that they could not serve their customers to their full satisfaction due to their power problem. Of 99 units, 61 (95.3%) and trade units and the rest 33 (94.3%) are industrial units.

Table 5

Number of Units Facing Problems Under Category II

S.No.	*Nature of Problem*	*Number of units today*					
		Trade	*%*	*Industry*	*%*	*Total*	*%*
1.	Attraction of customers by the competitors	54	83.4	22	62.9	76	76.8
2.	Customer's Dissatisfaction	61	95.3	33	94.3	94	95.0
3.	Loss of Business	38	59.4	16	45.7	54	54.6
4.	Increase in Overhead Expenses	27	42.2	34	97.1	61	61.6

Source: Primary Data 1992.

A businessman runs his business for his bread. Some interior island business units stated that they could not run their business after the sunset since the whole island weds with the darkness. They stated that they generally do half business. 54 units representing 55% of the total sample units facing power problem told that they loose their business only due to the total power cut. Of the 54 units, 38 (59.4%) are trade units and 16 (45.7%) are industrial units.

Increasing overhead expenses like unproductive wages and salaries, using light giving deices like candles, torch lights, and emergency lamps, refreshments, excess measures, less functions in more time etc. are another kind of problems contributing to the looses of the business. Sixty-one out of 99 sample units representing about 62% expressed that their overhead expenses are increasing due to the power problem. 61 units include 27 (42.2%) trade units and 34 (97.1%) industrial units. Comparing the trade units, the industrial units face more difficulties due to this power problem.

Category III

Rats, ants etc. also contribute their role a lot in making damage to the goods of the business units. They eat everything during night hours. The units find it very difficult to sell the packings ad packages spoiled by the rats, ants etc. Theft is another major problem due top the power cut. Since the territory has reached the saturation stage as far as the employment is concerned, number of theft incidents has been increasing. It is observed from the conversation with the respondents that their theft is happening especially at the time of power cut. Out of 99 respondents, 98 representing almost 100% stated that they have been experiencing such problems due to the power cut.

Suggestions

To remove the constraints of the power in A & N Islands, the following measures are suggested.

1. The A & N Administration may strengthen the existing structure by allocating more funds by appointing more qualified engineers etc. The Administration can increase the power tariff a little bit as suggested in Table 6. But in that case, the Administration should give a guarantee to their customers particularly to the business units that the power supply would be available for 24 hours in a day so that the business concerns can plan for their day to day development works without increasing the unproductive expenses.

Table 6

Suggested Power Tariff

S. No.	*Purpose/Tariff*	*Urban Area*		*Rural Area*	
			(In Rs.)		*(In Rs.)*
1.	For Domestic Purpose				
	Tariff per unit	1.00		0.75	
	Minimum Charge		10.00		6.00
2.	For Commercial Purpose				
	Tariff Per unit	1.50		1.00	
	Minimum Charge		40.00		25.00
3.	For Industrial Purpose				
	Tariff Per Unit	1.25		1.00	
	Minimum Charge		30.00		20.00

2. The A & N Administration may install some new generators in the business growth centres.
3. The A & N Administration can call the people from private sector for the establishment of power generating organisation in order to supply

power on the condition that there should not be power cut or shortage in the islands. In this regard, a political ad politics free committee should be formed and they may be entrusted with some special powers to control and advise the suggested private power organisation. The proposed committee should conduct a pilot studying in this regard. The total expenditure, revenue and other planning premises etc. should be taken into account.

4. The Local businessmen can be invited to install some common generators at the business growth centres. In such cases, the uninterrupted supply of diesel, other oil etc. may be assured by the Administration to the above said local businessmen having common generators. Subsidies, incentives, and other concessions may be granted without making further delay. If would be better to conduct a micro level survey to locate the growth centres.

Conclusion

Once the impediments in the path of business development are removed and an effective strategy is framed in the light of the above suggestions and adopted the activities of business will accelerate which will boost the economy of these islands.

References

1. Vepa Ram K "Small Industries" Vikas Publishing House Pvt. Ltd. New Delhi, 1983.
2. Rajavel N. "Problems and Prospects of Trade, Commerce and Industry in A & N Islands", Ph.D. Thesis, Kumaun University, Nainital, 1990.
3. Rajavel N. "Toys and Dolls Industry and its Prospects in the Bay Islands"

14

Problems of Industrial Cooperative Units in Bay Islands

Introduction

Cooperatives play a central role in the process of industrial development of the A & N Islands. In the past, peculiar social, economic, political and geographical condition of these islands restricted the emergence of creative industrial leadership. Consequently these islands, inspite of being very rich in natural resources, have remained industrially under developed. In the recent past, the government, cooperative department, commercial banks and cooperative banks have made efforts to create climate conductive to industrial entrepreneurship in these islands and as a result of which some industrial units have come up including cooperative units. Unfortunately, barring a few performances of these units, which could have otherwise proved to be pace- setters for others, have not been satisfactory and even some units are likely to become sick. At this crucial juncture, it is necessary to develop an insight into the problems being confronted by the units so that timely corrective actions may be taken and such plight may be checked. So a study was conducted to identify the major problems of the units as no such study was conducted earlier.

Study Area

A & N Islands consisting of 572 islands, rocks and hillocks, lie in the Bay of Bengal, is about 1200 Kms away from Madras and Calcutta have good potential of Natural Resources and offer better prospects for business activities with inhabitation of 35 islands. The details of these islands are described somewhere else by the author (Rajavel N 1992)

Industrial Cooperative Unit

There are 792 industrial units (as on 31-3-90) as per the report of the District Industries Centre, Port Blair. Of the total units, 36 units (as on 31-3-90) representing only 4.5% are the cooperative forms of business units. These cooperative units are engaged imprinting, binding works, hotel, shell crafts, bakery, tailoring etc. A sample of 15 units was taken for this study and was interviewed informally in order to elicit the problems faced by them and the identified problems are presented.

Problems

Industrial cooperative units, without doubt, have a very important role to play in the matter of the Bay Islands, economy. On the other hand they face a number of problems. The study reveals that the unit have faced numerous problem in the course of promotion and construction and at present they are contracting with the wide ranging operational problems which are given below.

Raw Materials

Procurement of raw materials of proper quality, in- adequate quantity at competitive prices is the most intricate problem faced by these units. Non – availability of raw materials, frequent interruptions in the availability of essential raw materials prevent the full capacity utilisation.

Transport and Communication

During the rainy season and unfavorable climate, these islands will be totally cut off from the mainland. So, these islands would face communication as well as transport problem and hence the units face the transport problem such as non- availability of transport and non-availability of space, cargo shut-out etc. As far as the internal transport is concerned, the demand or the lorries is heavy and the freight charges are also too much. This problem becomes acute during the days of ship arrival. Sometimes, even lorries many not be able though these units are willing to pay more charges.

Finance

Finance is the life- blood of business activities. The units are forced to borrow from the unorganized moneylenders in order to possess adequate working capital since thee financial assistance by the various institutional agencies including commercial banks often falls much short of their requirements.

Technology

Majority of the units have production methods of low technological level. Modern techniques are totally absent in these units. This has resulted in their continued low productivity and poor quality of the goods.

Market

The industrial cooperative units of this territory face the problems in order to market their product. They find it difficult to export their products to the mainland due to the transport problems, lack of market, information etc. Prevailing demand and supply position in different places of market can be known only through an effective marketing information which is totally absent in these islands. This is one of the major problems facing the units. There are regulated markets in the A & N Islands. That's why these units suffer form un-remunerative prices for their products. These units suffer from inadequacy of market research and good information system.

Other problems

Non – availability of skilled workers and drivers, unfavorable climate, intolerable delay on the part of different officers, indifferent attitude of the officials, frequent power cuts and its consequences (Rajavel 1992) and competition of the small –scale units and medium- scale units are the other problems facing the units.

Suggestions

The following measures are suggested to solve the problems and for the overall development of the industrial cooperative units.

1. The industrial cooperative units should be given adequate degree of priority in the allocation pattern of essential, but scarce, raw materials and equipments. These units should be encouraged to replace their out moded equipment with that incorporating and up-to-date technology, and facilities and incentives should be provided wherever required.

2. Unnecessary delays on the part of the different officers are to be totally avoided. Different officers involved in the industrial development should meet at least once in a month at a common place. The industrialists, entrepreneurs etc. are also to be invite on the day. Their problems are to be discussed and the necessary sanctions must be granted on the same day.

3. With full advantages of changing technique of production, dispensation of technical knowledge to the units should form an

essential element of the overall strategy. A system of integrated credit, i.e., long-term credit and short-term credit is to be made available at the rate of interest, which these units can bare.

4. The A & N Administration may procure the finished products of the industrial units at a fixed rate and those products may be exported to the mainland. For this purpose of marketing the products, the administration establishes sales counters at different places preferably in cities and towns of the mainland.

Conclusion

Once the impediments in the path of the industrial development in A & N islands are removed and an effective strategy is framed in the light of the above suggestions and adopted, the industrial activities will boost the economy of these islands.

15

Management of Cooperative Education and Training in a Islands

Introduction

The term "cooperation" mans living, thinking and working together. But in Commerce Education, it means a special form of Business Organisation with the merits and advantages of the cooperative form of business; they adopted different methods and techniques in the field of cooperation. The Commerce experts, economists, socialists etc, believe that it is the best form of organisation in which there is no scope of being exploited by middlemen or others and with a lot scope of satisfaction, standard of living, promoting the poors, self, help, for no partiality etc. Hence, number of committees, commissions, centres, institutes etc. conducted different studies, surveys on cooperation in order to use this golden tool in each and every field of economic development. The success and failure of such techniques and movement fully depend on the Cooperative Education and Training of its members, organizers, officers, auditors, inspectors and employees as a whole. But such education and training, to the extent what the author has understood, is not imparted fully in A & N Islands though there is a full-fledged Cooperative Department with an excellent network system of Cooperation and Cooperative Movement in these islands. So, an attempt has been made in this paper to give the importance of Cooperative Education and Training to high light the management of curriculum of Cooperative Education and Training and the need of such education in these islands.

A & N Islands

A & N Islands consisting of 572 islands, rocks and hillocks, lie in the Bay of Bengal, is about 1200 kms. away from Chennai and Calcutta, have good potential; of Natural Resources and offer better prospects for the Cooperative form of Business Organisations in all economic activities with inhabitation of 38 islands. The details of these islands are described somewhere else by the author. (Rajavel. N. 1992)

Cooperative Education Training

Cooperative education is a very broad term, which cannot be defined by a single line or two. The importance of Cooperative Education & Training is realised much before the cooperative movement and societies. Many eminent scholars like Sir Fredrick Nicholson (1895), Dr. M.S. Swaminathan (1973) and like had stressed the importance of the education and training. The ICA Commission (1966) recommended "all cooperative societies should make provisions for the education of their members, officers, and employees and of general public, in the principles and techniques of cooperation, both economic and democratic". The Cooperative Education develops the mental faculties, increase the knowledge and sharpen the intellect, broaden the vision etc, and the training gives the practical shape. So the Cooperative Education can be defined as the conscious preparation of individual, members, officers another employees with the full knowledge of Cooperation, Principles and Practices of Cooperation, Management of Cooperatives, Systems and Techniques of Cooperation, organisation etc. The cooperative training means the art of preparing the cooperative educated, existing employees of the cooperative units as a practical cooperative leader through practice by placing them on- the – job. The Cooperative Education and Training are fully responsible for the success and failure of the system.

Present Situation in A & N Islands

When other things remain unchanged, the Cooperative Unions of the State are fully responsible for imparting the Cooperative Education & Training. In A & N Islands, there is a full – fledged Cooperative Department And Cooperative Union with 440 cooperative societies with 52063 members. Of the 440 societies, 376 with 47470 members are in Andaman District and 64 with the membership strength of 4493 are in Nicobar District. Number of Cooperative Societies, number of members. , Amount of working capital and reserve fund is given in Table No. 1. It is evident from the table that he number of societies is increasing by marking a significant growth in the years 1992 and 1991 at the rate of 8.1% a and 7.8% respectively. The table also recorded a commendable growth in 1994 from the base year 1990, that is, about 5 times these islands. Moreover all types of cooperative societies are functioning in these islands particulars about which are given in Table 2. All these societies are progressing at a satisfactory level.

Need

But how many employees, workers, members of such societies have full knowledge on cooperation? And how many of them have been trained? Are the important points to be considered? In almost all the cooperative societies, majority of the staff are untrained. One-way or other they fully depend on others as far as the knowledge and practical solutions on cooperative management are concerned. At present, the employees of the Cooperative Department are sent to the mainland cities namely Chennai, Calcutta, and New Delhi etc. for getting Cooperative Education and training. The employees of the cooperative societies or units of these islands could not think of going for training to the mainland due to economic reasons.

So, it is very essential to provide Cooperative Education and Training to all the members, employees of all cooperative units. Moreover, the education and training should be made compulsory by the department and the government to all the office bearers of the existing cooperative societies and members of the cooperatives, which will be registered in future. So, there must be a separate institute in the A & N Islands to provide and impart the cooperative education and training which is the need of this hour.

Management

Management of curriculum of the Cooperative Education and Training in these islands is a very crucial point to be considered. Though the Cooperative Education and Training are the same in all over the country in A & N Islands a special management is required. This is an education in responsibilities, duties, and accountabilities and in human relations. In these, far flung islands, people from different regions and religions, cultures, and faith are living without any difference of opinion. So, the trainees or the participants should necessarily have knowledge about the environmental conditions, population characters, economic conditions of the different classes of population, resources etc. of these islands. Just one cannot introduce the same curriculum of the Cooperative Education and Training in the mainland in A & N Islands also. Due care must be taken while framing the curriculum/ syllabi for such education in these islands by providing the weightage to the above features without which, certainly, the system will wed with failure. So, as a highlight, the following outline of the curriculum is being recommended by the author in this piece of work.

FOR ONE YEAR DIPLOMA

Theory/ Practical / Seminar	*Name of the Paper/ Project Report*
(A) Theory Papers	1. Economics of A & N Islands
	2. Population Studies of A & N Islands
	3. Principles of Cooperation
	4. Management of Cooperatives
	5. Principles of Book Keeping and Auditing
(B) Practical Training	1. One Month On – The – Job Training
	2. Submission of report about the Training
(C) Seminar & Workshop	1. Seminar at the last Saturday of every month with a minimum of 6 programmes
	2. Workshop once in 4 months with a minimum of 2 programmes.

FOR TWO YEARS DIPLOMA

Theory/ Practical / Seminar	*Name of the Paper/ Project Report*
(A) Theory Papers	1. Economics of A & N Islands
	2. Population Studies of A & N Islands
	3. Fundamentals of Business Organisation
	4. Principles of Accounting
	5. Mercantile Law including Negotiable Instrument Act
	6. Principles and Practice of Cooperation
	7. Management of Cooperatives
	8. Govt. and Cooperatives including Cooperative Legislations
	9. Cooperative Auditing
	10. Income Tax for Cooperatives
(B) Practical Training	1. Two months on-the-job training in different Cooperatives- one month each at the end of Every year
	2. Submission of detailed report about the On-the-job training
	3. Submission of a project report about a Possible line of business in the form of Cooperative.
(C) Seminar & Workshop	1. Seminar at the last Saturday of every month With a minimum of 6 programmes
	2. Workshop once in 4 months with a minimum of 2 programmes.

(D) Viva – Voce	1. Every student/Participant will be asked to Appear before the eminent scholars/ Academicians for viva – voce test.

Provision for internal Assessment marks, marks for practical problem solving methods etc. are to be included. One year and two years Diploma Courses are to be considered as qualifications for the different posts in the Cooperative Department/ Units etc. Since this paper gives only the highlight of the project of Cooperative Education and Training, a detailed discussion may be held to finalise the course with the author.

Suggestions

1. An Institute for the Cooperative Education and Training should immediately be started in the A & N Islands. If it is already included in the Five Year Planning Proposal, then the delay in starting the Institute should be avoided and steps to start the Institute are to be taken.
2. The curriculum for the Cooperative Education and Training in A & N Islands should be specially designed with the consultation of the Experts and Academicians.
3. First al the present employees of the Department and various units should be trained over a period 2 – 3 years along with the limited number of fresh candidates separately. Then the new courses should be stared in the light of the above highlights.
4. Studies should be conducted or encourages on the problems of the Cooperative and Cooperative Movement in these far flung islands and the possible future prospects must be explored.
5. Intensive advertisement and publicity should be made about the cooperative principles, concession and subsidies available to the cooperatives etc.
6. Compulsion must be made that the person who got the Cooperative Education and Training must only be granted permission to start the cooperatives and such person should be appointed in the Cooperative Department and units in the different posts.

Conclusion

At the present situation, Cooperative Education and Training is absolutely essential tour A & N Islands. Cooperative sector in A& N Islands is at present having a lot of projects and can be used as a very important media for the overall economic development of these resourceful islands. For that purpose, the effective system of education and training is to be installed in the light of the above discussion and once it is installed, the Cooperative Movement will, definitely, be a successful method in these islands.

Table No. 1

Cooperatives and its progress in Andaman and Nicobar Islands

Year	*Societies*		*Members*		*Reserve Fund*		*Working Capital*	
	Nos.	*%*	*Nos.*	*%*	*Nos.*	*%*	*Nos.*	*%*
1990	409	–	50.1	–	124.8	–	2198.9	–
1991	422	3.2	51.4	2.8	298.1	138.9	2429.9	10.5
1992	442	8.1	51.8	3.6	299.1	139.7	2590.2	17.8
1993	427	4.4	52.0	3.8	299.4	139.9	2598.5	18.2
1994	440	7.8	52.1	4.0	675.0	440.9	1419.2	(–)35.5

Source: Primary Data

Note: % is calculated by taking 1990 as the base year.

Table no. 2

Types of cooperatives and its members in A & N Islands

S.No. Name	*Societies (Nos.)*	*Members (Nos.)*	*Share Capital (Rs) (in Lakhs)*
1. Agricultural Credit	44	16535	32.52
2. Non-Agricultural Credit	19	2111	2.98
3. Consumer	37	20465	14.30
4. Marketing	35	3640	8831
5. Plantation	26	795	1.82
6. Industrial	42	1408	10.74
7. Housing	53	1390	22.82
8. Milk/Poultry/Fisheries	76	2442	11.18
9. Transport	29	497	1.12
10. Others	79	2780	7.25
Total	440	52063	193.04

Source: Basic Statistics 1994.

16

Management of Change

Introduction

The study of organizational behaviour is very important in every organisation. Organisational Behaviour (OB) means, a field of study that investigates the impacts that individuals, groups and structure have behaviour within the organisation, for the purpose of applying such knowledge towards improving organisation effectiveness. OB is an applied field. It applies the knowledge gained about individuals; groups and the effect of structure on behaviour towards the need of making organisations work more effectively. The study of OB includes the study of motivation, leader behaviour and power, interpersonal communication, group structure and process, attitude of development and perception, change process, conflict, job design and work stress. Of all, "Change" is taken in this paper for the discussion since it is important because "Change" changes the attitude of human resources, the whole performance quickly and the entire literature of the OB.

What is "Change"?

The dictionary meaning of the term "Change" is "alteration". But the term "Change" here means making things different. It includes two more elements namely, Change Intervention and Change Agent. Change Intervention is a planned action to make things different. Change agent is a person or are persons who act(s) as catalyst(s) and assumes the responsibility or responsibilities for managing the change process.

So, change may be defined as, any variation or deviation, occurred naturally or willingly made with a plan of action by a person or persons who will be made responsible for such variation or alterations, from the exciting state.

Change Agents

The change agents may be managers or non – managers, employees or organisation or out-side consultants. If management decides to introduce a change, if it is a major one, the management may hire the service of out-side consultants to provide advice and assistance. The service of the outside consultant has drawbacks because they usually have an inadequate understanding of the organisation's history, culture, operation, process and procedures, and personnels. The out- side consultants may prove to initiate more drastic changes. This may be of a benefit or disadvantage because they do not have to live with a consequence after the change is implemented. So, in order to avoid this type of hurdles internal staff specialists or managers are to be considered as "Change Agents" because they may be thoughtful and possibly cautious since they must live with the consequences of their actions. Hence, here my view and opinion is that the outside consultants should not be involved in the "Change Process" and the internal staff specialists should be considered as "Change Agents".

Why "Change"?

This is the biggest question that whether "change" is needed for a smooth going concern. The answer is yes. The change is needed for the following reasons:

(a) To survive in the present competitive business world.

(b) To increase production by adopting new technology such as installing the new computerized machines.

(c) To Maintain a status in the business world

(d) To improve its market share

(e) To serve the society best through introducing new products, new usages of the existing products and good quality products at reasonable price.

(f) To give enough opportunities to the dedicated employees for promotions and new positions etc.

(g) To face competitions etc.

Do Employees Resist "Change"?

Another questions to be answered is that when a change is introduced; will it be welcomed or accepted by all employees? The answer is certainly not. Though not all, the majority of the people will resist "change". Here people refer the employees of the organisation. Main reason for the resistance is the attitude of the people that not to work in a new circumstance. They get satisfaction at the level at the salary, at the knowledge, at the control what they have at present. Some people like and accept change because they want to go themselves, to have more technological knowledge and top occupy a position in the organisation. The reasons for the resistances are given below.

1. Fear of Loss of Employment and Unableness

Generally people resist change only on the fear of loss of employment. They also have a sort of negative attitudes towards change. They think if change takes place that they may be thrown out of the job. If for example, the introduction for world processors means that departmental secretaries will have to learn to operate this new pieces of equipments, some of the secretaries may fear that they may lose their jobs, some other as may fear that they will be unable to do so. They m ay, therefore, develop negative attitude towards working with word processors or behave dysfunctionally is required to use them.

2. Envy

The quality of being jealous is another reason to resist change. For example, in an organisation the superior may be less educated than his subordinate and if the organisation brings change and thereby the subordinate as likely going to be promoted either to equal status or part of the superior due to jealousy. This state of affairs is also visible among people who are working in the same status.

3. Fear of Personal Loss

The other cause of resistance is fear of personal loss of something already possessed. Change threatens the 'investment' one has already made in the status. The people have invested more in the current system, the more resistant they tend to be toward change. The fears of loss of status, money, authority, friendships, personal convenience, or other benefits they value are the reasons for the resistance to change.

4. Fear of Transfer

People resist change due to fear of transfer also. A kind of fear " I may be transferred" occurs if there is any "change" in the organisation attributes to the resistance. For example, if an organisation brings diversification in its structures, some of the senior officers may be made in charge of the branches for which they are to be transferred. So, there will be a strong resistance on the part of the officers who enjoyed the privileges of the present employment, place etc.

Change Process

Without resistance, no organisation can bring "Change". When resistance to change is seen as dysfunctional, what action can be taken?

Reducing resistances to change can best be understood only after understanding the "Change Process" Change process are in three stages. They are:

1. Unfreezing
2. Movement or Change itself and
3. Refreezing

They are shown in the following diagram:

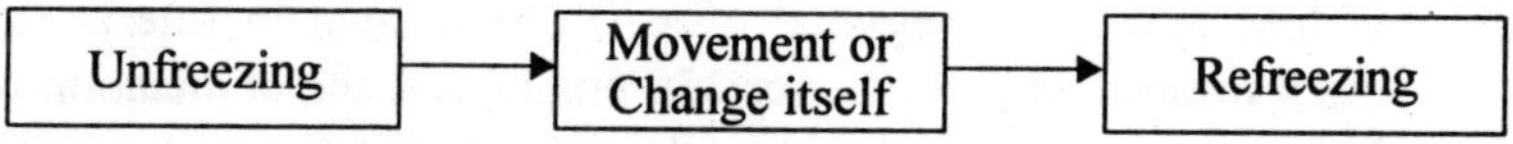

1. Unfreezing State

This is the first stage. Unfreezing means, the activity of making one's brain vacuum. That is the people should not have any negative approach in their mind or in other words that are prepared to see the things with the positive approach when "change" is made. This stage may be created by adopting anyone of the methods – Demeaning, Physical Removal, Reward or Punishment. For example, if change is made and people resist with strong negative approach, under such circumstances, the change agents can pursue frequently the merits of "change" as a reply to their doubts, questions or approaches. This is called Demeaning. If a particular person makes the whole group unrest, he may be removed from the service. However, this is subjected to other circumstances also. Or he may be treated with some monetary benefits or promotions (reward) in order to shut his mouth. If management and maximum number of employees feel that someone is hindering the development of change and also if the situation says clearly that he can not be removed from the service, then the person may be punished by the way of demotion, cut the increments etc. By doing so, the group may be prepared to accept the "change".

2. Change Itself or Movement Stage

This is the second right stage in which change can be implemented. The proposed change is to be very carefully and slowly introduced by the change agents. This state takes organisation to a new state. Once the change agent comes to this stage, he should be very careful, while implementing, that the people should not take the agent to the first stage.

3. Refreezing Stage

This is the last stage. Here, the change agent has to take all the necessary steps, which are all acceptable in order to make the change permanent. This is stabilizing a change intervention by balancing driving and restraining forces.

An Example:

The management of a large cloth-manufacturing company decided to reorganize its marketing functioning in Tamil Nadu State. The company had five divisional offices located in Madras, Chidambaram, Elleri, Kattumannar Koil and in Thanjavur. The decision was made to consolidate the divisions into single regional office to be located in Elleri. The recognition meant transferring over 330 employees; the elimination of some duplicated managerial position and the institution of a new hierarchy of command. As a matter of fact, a move of this magnitude was difficult to keep secret. The rumor of its occurrence preceded the announcement by several months. The decision itself was made unilaterally. It came from executive officers, Madras. Those people affected had no say whatsoever in the choice for those in Chidambaram or Kattumannar Koil who may have disliked the decision and the consequences, the problems inherent in transferring to another town, pulling youngsters out of school, making new friends, having new co- workers, the undergoing the reassignment of responsibilities – their only recourse was to quit. This example will be used to illustrate the unfreezing, movement and the refreezing model.

Management

Management can expect employees the resistance to the consolidation. To deal with that resistance, the management can use any of the methods of demeaning, rewards etc. to make employees to accept the change. For instance, increases in pay can be offered to those accept the transfer. The company can pay very liberal moving expenses. The company may offer low cost mortgage funds to allow employees to buy new homes in Elleri. Of course, management may choose to unfreeze acceptance of the status quo by removing restraining forces. Each employees concerns apprehensions could be heard and clarified specially. Assuming that most of fears are unjustified, the counselor could assure the employees that there was nothing to fear and then to demonstrate through tangible evidence that restraining forces are unwarranted. In case the resistance is extremely high, management may have to resort to both reducing resistance and increasing the attractiveness of the alternate if the unfreezing is to be successful. Once unfreezing has been accomplished, the change itself can be implemented.

How to Overcome Resistance to Change?

The change agents should have to adopt some tactics to overcome the resistance to change. The tactics are listed and discussed below:

1. Communication
2. Education
3. Participation
4. Negotiation
5. Manipulation and Cooptation
6. Facilitation and Support
7. Coercion

1. Communication

This is the simple tactic, which will impress many people to reduce the resistance to change. If change is communicated to all levels of management, they will develop an ego of 'I am consulted and I am also regarded.' So to some extent through communication, the resistance to change can be controlled. If the employees receive full facts and get any misunderstandings cleared up, the full resistance will subside.

2. Education

Resistance can be handled and overcome through education – one-on-one discussion, memos, group discussions, group presentations or reports. The management will have to educate the employees about the importance, necessities, and advantages of the proposed change. Though all do not understand atleast the understood people will convince the rest.

3. Participation

This method is just like putting the name of the troublemaker in village in the invitation card of some general celebration and occasions of the village. Once if the name is placed in the invitation card, the troublemaker will never create trouble rather he will work hard to make the function successful. It is difficult for individual to resist change decision in which they participated prior to making a change. Assuming that participants have the experience to make a meaningful contribution, their involvement can reduce resistant, obtain commitment and increase the quality of change decision.

4. Negotiation

This is another way to handle the resistance to change. This is just like offering some rewards, which will meet the needs of a person who resist. Particularly if the resistance is more and centered in a few powerful individuals, as referred before, a specific reward package can be negotiated that will meet their individual needs.

5. Manipulation and Cooptation

Here manipulation refers the activity of making or created false rumors as untrue threat. That is twisting and distorting facts to make them appear more attracting, with holding undesirable information to get employees to accept change are all the examples of manipulation. Once if the employees come to know that the threat is actually untrue, they will accept, with full heart, the change. Cooptation, on the other hand, is some sort of manipulation with participation . This is just like purchasing the leader of the resistance group by giving them a key role in the change decision. The leaders advise is sought, not to seek a better decision, but to get their endorsement. This method is, no doubt, inexpensive but the top management level will have to tolerate a lot.

6. Facilitation and Support

The management can offer a range of supportive efforts to reduce the resistance. When employees fear and anxiety are high, employee counseling and therapy, new skills training or a short period leave of absence may facilitate adjustment.

7. Coercion

This is last method. This is a kind of application of direct threats or force upon employees who resist. The examples of coercion are the direct threats of transfer, loss of promotions, negative performances evaluations or the poor letter of recommendations.

Conclusion

As a conclusion, the change for every organisation is absolutely necessary to live in the business world, to retain the market share, to compete the competitors, to serve the individuals, society at large, better, to give more and more opportunities to the dedicated employees by the way of promotion, new position etc. Change is to be introduced very carefully and slowly in stages by stages. Lazy cum inefficient will definitely resists. They will have to be very carefully handled. The resistance to change may be overcomed through education, communication, rewards, manipulation, cooptation, and coercion,. If it is necessary some facilities and support may be given to the employee of the organisation. Even if there is any resistance, the resistors are to be treated with threats of transfer, cutting their increments and likes. After adopting all those techniques and tactics, still if it is impossible to control the resistor or resistors they are to removed from the service compromisely.

17

Need for Air Subsidy in the Economic Development of Andaman and Nicobar Islands

Introduction

India is still considered as a developing country. This is due to many reasons such as increasing population, low per-capita real income, poor Infrastructural facilities, under utilisation of resources, barriers in the labour mobilization, Mass poverty, high cost of living, absolute methods of production, lack of skilled personnel, lack of entrepreneurial talent, non-economic factors like favoritism, nepotism and corruption etc. economic development requires efficient, dedicated and clean administration and management at all levels. The political, cultural and social developments have no meaning without the economic development and prosperity. There are a lot of factors responsible for the development of our country. Of all, transport is the main and vital factor. This paper is restricted to only the role of transport in economic development and further restricted to our Green Paradise, picturesque, enchanting beautiful and resourceful A & N Islands.

A & N Islands

A & N Islands, situated in the Bay of Bengal are surrounded by Burma, Thailand, Malaysia and Indonesia. The islands constitute the most isolated part of India Union, stretching in North South Direction, separated from the Mainland of India vast stretches of sea. The Andaman groups of islands are separated from Nicobar Group of Islands by 10-degree channel. This territory, comprising an area of 8293 square kilometers in a group of picturesque islands. Port Blair, the capital of this Bay Islands is connected with the Mainland by both sea and air routes. The population of A & N

Islands is 2.80,661 as per the census year 1991. The rate of growth is 48.7% over the previous census year. The seat of Administration is situated in Port Blair City.

Economic Status

Only from the recent past, these Islands witness some development, which can be counted for economic development. Number of industrial units, trade units, commercial units, travel units started increasing by showing a growing trend at a lower rate. The Chamber of Commerce and Industry Associations of Small Scale Units and trade associations have been contributing their possible efforts to the growth of these islands. But all such valuable efforts couldn't bring the expected result due to some unsolvable problems at our end which are pushing down the economy of the A & N island to the infant stage status. However, such unsolvable problems can be solved by the Govt. of India, if desired.

Ingredients of the Economy

Each and every aspects and transactions is no doubt, responsible for the economic development of this territory. Of all, the major and main ingredients are Agriculture, Trade, Commerce, Industry and Tourism. Agriculture is the backbone of our Indian Economic System since it is the supplier of food. Industry plays an important role by providing employment opportunity, meeting consumer needs, help in resource utilization, accelerating economic growth, mobilizing manpower, promoting self-employment. As far as the trade is concerned, the domination of internal import trade is the more than the internal export trade. But sill the trade plays a very vital role by mobilizing and transferring the goods and services from the different parts of the mainland to these islands and from one island to another island. In a research work on Problems and Prospects of trade, Commerce and Industry in A & N Islands by Dr. N. Rajavel HOD Commerce JNRM, Port Blair (Me) Trade Activity is named as "LIFE GIVING ASPECT." Commerce i.e. transports banking, storage, insurance and advt. Contributes its share to some extends. Tourism, a smokeless industry is also one of the major ingredients of the economy. Though it is in infant stage it stretches its arms by inviting a large number of visitors. The role of Trade, Commerce, Industry and Tourism in the economic development of A & N Islands are the excellent and needy topics for Seminar. It is left to the concerned departments for the organization of Seminar.

Role of Transport

Transport plays a vital role because the quick transports help in opening up remote and inaccessible regions, promotes labour mobility, protects the market, helps in the movement of raw materials, fuels, machinery, finished goods, promote industries and widening the peoples out look which is very important factor. For accelerating the economic growth particularly in A & N Islands, it is not merely the physical resources which are required also progressive out look of the people indicating urge for economic uplift and ready responsiveness to new suggestions. In fact, the modern out look of the people is important determinant of economic growth.

Prospects

Once A & N Islands was coined as " KALAPANI" a black water. But it is no more KALAPANI. No doubts, this territory gains a lot of developments in every field. But the rate of growth is very low. What do we NOT have in these islands? We have everything here. Why should we depend upon Mainland for everything? We can make the Mainland to depend upon land, it is totally wrong. Even in the available land what have been produced and exported to the mainland so far? Now what is going here is that we send all goods at raw level to the mainland and we buy he the finished goods from there. For ex. We send betelnut Arecaunut (supari) at raw level but we buy the finished products of the Arecaunut line sugandh supari, scented supari, seeval supari, pan parag etc. We send coconuts but we buy coconut oil and oil cake from the mainland and like this many products at its raw level are sent to mainland which is against the principles of paper, vegetables and like can be produced and manufactured here itself. There are no toys and dolls industry in these islands at small-scale level, which has excellent market potentiality both in mainland and abroad. Casavarina plantation, Mango plantation, Eucalyptus plantation, Coconut plantation, Cashew plantation, and Arecaunut plantation show encouraging results. All these cash crop plantations will certainly increase the income of territory in long run by promoting number of small- scale units. This territory has historical resources for tourism industry. By its multiplier effect, the tourism industry helps in increasing the economic development. Hence, this territory has excellent potentiality and prospects for all the economic activities.

Pitiable Conditions

How the people of A & N Islands are living here, just can't be told in fifteen minutes. People living here on the principles of comparative disadvantages. This is like that we have everything here but we can't enjoy. We have butter but we spend more money to buy ghee. We have milk but we spend more money to buy curd. We have eyes but we can't see. We have strength the legs are under locked to run. We have a lot to eat and the mouth is on plaster and so on. These islands have excellent industrialists, traders, commercialists, and experts but they can't show their full capacities. We have all factors of production but lack of cheep and quickest mode of transportation i.e. Air Transport. The people of these islands have to pay huge amount on essential items and on urgent health care. Our businessmen can't take a quick decision on the matters related to their units. Our journalists and press intellectual can't go and come from the mainland for their routine development. When this is the pitiable conditions of these pillars of the roof of A & N Islands, one can just think about the position of middle class and lower class (on the basis of income) general public. The problems are more acute in inter islands. Quick movements between the islands and from the islands to the mainland are almost very difficult which may encourage delayed postal marriages only due to the want of bearable and quickest mode of transport. The present cost of air travel is heavy, unbearable, intolerable, unacceptable and highly objectionable to the people of A & N Islands. Besides the heavy cost of Air Travel, the allied cost of expenditure adds fuel to the burning fire.

Need for Subsidy

For the economic activity of business, raw materials, finished products, manpower, capital, technical know-how suggestions are the important aspects. They are to be mobilized to bring development. Now at present subsidy is granted by Govt. of India upto 90% of the total transport cost. But it is restricted to only between ports to ports. Machinery Transportation for the units, Goods and services to the commercial and trade units, transports for the tourism units even between port to port are not eligible for transport subsidy. Also no subsidy is granted for the transportation of raw materials and finished goods by air. If the important aspects are continuously mobilized without any interruption, it is highly hopped that the big vessel economic development of A & N islands will certainly move fast of its own. But the vessel is at present in stagnant level. It needs some push and pull as in the case of a big ships which placed on route by push and pull by a small Bhalshali boat which I mean to refer here is as subsidy. In Particular Air Subsidy.

Stress for Air Subsidy

Though the subsidy for both the transports is needed, there is an urgent need for air subsidy to the people of these islands because the air transport is the only quickest mode of travel available like rail and road. For health reason, social reasons less availability of other modes of travel, to give quick transportation service to the people etc. But A & N Islands is also one of the Backward Area like NER notified by the Govt. of India. A & N Islands is also industrially backward area identified by the Govt. of India and in particular, the Car Nicobar is declared by the Govt. Of India as No Industry Area. On a comparison, the NER has all sorts of facilities as far as the transports and travels are concerned. They have rail transport, road transports etc. but for the people of A & N island only one mode of transport i.e. slow going ship transport is available besides the heavy unbearable cost of air travel. Moreover, these islands have historical importance to attract the tourists of all categories. Hence, no one can justify that the air subsidy should not be granted to the people of A & N Islands.

Air Traffic

Air traffic between this territory and the mainland records a vital importance. About 40,000 passengers are traveling annually in each sector, about 4,50,000 kgs cargo about 1,50,000 kgs mails are carried annually between the islands and the mainland each sector. This is besides the ship traffic. This is an excellent evidence for the importance of Air Transport to these islands and the need for air subsidy.

Air Fare

At present the airfare between Port Blair and Chennai is Rs. 5,920 and between Port Blair and Calcutta is Rs. 5,850. The same was Rs. 3727 and Rs. 3,687 as on 31.05.95. The rate of increase in the airfare is about into three parts namely basic fare, passenger service fee, and internal air travel tax representing 85%, 2% and 13% respectively.

Suggestions

The following measures are offered in the form of suggestions to overcome the problems due to the heavy cost of Air Travel and in the matter of granting air subsidy.

1. The existing transport subsidy may be extended to SSI units to bring the machinates from the mainland. The same subsidy may be granted to the SSI units from the place purchase of raw materials to the place of the unit in these islands and from the place of production factory to the place of market both in islands and in mainland without counting the ports.

2. Transport subsidy for the service sector when they purchase and brought goods and services into these islands may also be considered for the promotions of economic activities in this territory. The govt. of India may introduce a scheme a sir transport subsidy for cargo traffic also.
3. It is highly suggested that the govt. of India may kindly grant a passenger air subsidy of 30% of the total air fare of all air traffic sector of SER, A & N Islands as is done in case of NER (or)
4. The A & N Administration may fix the air fare by taking all factors into consideration for (a) ISALANDERS and (b) for OTHERS as is done in the case of islands ship transport. The difference between the fare fixed by the Admn. And fare fixed by the Airlines authorities may be borne by the local govt./Central Govt.. This is purely in the interest of the public, SSI units, trade, commerce and Industry and Tourism. At present, the Govt. of India grants subsidy on ship passengers traffic on each classes say bunk class, cabin class etc. if the same % of subsidy is granted to the Air Traffic also the air fare will be reduced to 40% to 50%. (or)
5. An autonomous body of Island Air Service in the name of BAY ISLAND AIRLINES may be established/started in Port Blair, under the management of a dedicated officer. The proposed organisation may buy initially ONE/TWO aircrafts for Mainland-Island Service and ONE/TWO helicopters for the inter-island services. Daily one trip to Chennai and one trip to Calcutta is suggested. It is also suggested to have more number of trips to these places at the time of demand.
6. A & N Administration or the Govt. of India may fix its own fare by diverting the subsidy granted to the ship transport to the proposed BY ISLANDS AIRLAINES. The fare can be moderately fixed at a rate which will be equal to even less than 70% of the present fare with the help of Management Accounting Techniques such as Margin of Safety Analysis, Cost –Profit- Volume Analysis, Ratio Analysis etc. by taking some bounties from the Govt. of India.
7. Of course, initially the new proposed island airlines may have problems in manning and maintenance of the crafts (which may be managed effectively on the principles of the management by objectives and the management by exception) to overcome that problem, the present operating airlines may be entrusted with the work of manning and maintenance, if necessary.

8. Giving suggestions and criticizing the same may be very easy but how difficult it will be felt only when such suggestions are an application. Hence, it is suggested to constitute a politics free high power committee consisting of dedicated officers, experts, and representatives of the trade, commerce and industry associations etc. and authorities of the existing airlines to study the feasibility of the suggestions by taking everything in a right angle. The committee may be directed to draw/ frame a constructive strategy on the systems of ISLAND AIRLINES, and on the grant of air subsidy by the Govt. of India, and possibility of fixing air fare for Islanders and others.

Conclusion

Hence, I conclude, that A & N Islands is rich in resources and they are to be exploited fully. Agriculture, Plantations, Cash Crops, SSI units, Commerce and Trade Units and Tourism have excellent PROSPECTS and are the important ingredients of economic development of A & N Islands. Raw materials, finished products, man power, suggestions, Technical know-how and finance are to be mobilized. The public face is intolerable and unbearable problems due to the heavy cost of quickest mode of travel i.e. Air Travel. The Govt. of India is kindly granted that Air Subsidy to NER by leaving the SER (A & N Islands) though the people of A & N Islands are the suffers due to the want of quickest modes of travels. Though the people of A & N Islands as is given in for the NER. If a constructive strategy or policy is framed in the light of the above suggestions and discussion and implemented through dedicated and really qualified officers on the expert's advises/suggestions, I hope that the people this SER (A & N Islands) at a large will highly be benefited increasing by their standard of living and certainly the ECONOMY OF A & N ISLAND WILL BE DEVELOPED,

18

An Empirical Study on Workings of the Traders in Diglipur Island

Introduction

Trade both internal and international gives a country advantageous to the better industrialisation and standard of living and thereby it increases the economic development of the country. But the Trade and its extent of effectiveness fully depend upon the entrepreneurs the country/region has, the technology they are capable of using, the risk they are prepared to bear, opportunities they are ready to search and accept. The success of an entrepreneur depends fully on the qualities required to innovate, start a new enterprise, accept the challenge and bear the risk. Trade activities as a whole, is a Sine- quo non-of economic progress It is one of the important means to improve the economy. Andaman and Nicobar Islands are fully Blessed with the resources, but the growth of Trade in A & N islands is not even at the satisfactory level.. The people of these islands fully depends upon the Mainland for all goods both essential, constructions, luxurious, durable and non-durable goods. Less education or lack of education on the part of the entrepreneurs is one of the main reasons for such slow growth. Diglipur Island is one of the very important islands of this territory and is a fast growing Trade Centre. Major portion of cultivation is carried out in this island. Keeping in view of trade entrepreneur as the key point, a study has been conducted to analyse their workings in the Diglipur Island as no study has been conducted earlier. Since the Diglipur Island is having the potentiality for the Agricultural Products, for attracting the Tourists and thereby the establishment of Tourism Industry, to reduce the unemployment problems etc., this island is considered economically important place and hence the Diglipur Island is taken for the study.

Bay Islands

The Bay Islands (A & N Islands) situated in the Bay of Bengal and it is located between 6 degree and 14 degree of NL and 92 degree and 94 degree of EL. This is surrounded by Burma, Thailand, Malaysia and Indonesia and it constitute the most isolated place part of Indian Union, stretching in North South direction, separated from Indian mainland by vast stretches of sea. Andaman group of islands is separated from the Nicobar group of islands by the boisterous 10-degree channel, which is about 155 kms. wide and 400 fathoms deep. This territory comprising an area of 8293 Sq. kms. is a group of islands. Of the total number of islands in this territory, only 38 islands are inhabited. Port Blair, the capital of this union territory, is connected by both sea and air routes with the mainland of India. The sea distance between Port Blair - Chennai; Port Blair -Calcutta and Port Blair- Vishakapatanam is 1190 kms., 1255 kms., and 1200 kms. respectively. This territory is divided in 2 Districts, 3 Divisions, 7 Tehsils and 8 Regions (Rajavel 1990).

Diglipur Islands

Diglipur Island is situated in North Andaman Island group. It is a separate Island. It is fully inhabited island. It is well connected with other islands by seaways. Recently the Andaman and Nicobar Administration has been seriously planning helicopter service to this resourceful island. The different places inside the island are connected by roads. The sea distance between Diglipur and Port Blair 165 kms; Mayabunder and Diglipur is 28 kms. As per the Census year 2001, the total population of the Diglipur Island is 42,880 consisting of 52.74% Males and 47.26% of Females. The literacy rate in the Diglipur Island is 74.98%. The density of the population has been increasing every year.

The status of the Population is Rural. The settlers of this island is mainly Bengalis, Malayalies, Tamilians and Telugu. The main occupation of these people is cultivation of paddy, vegetables, and fruits. The census villages in the Diglipur island is about 42. the average population of Diglipur Islands is about 600 per village. Kalipur, in this island is a beautiful sandy beach has been developed as a tourist complex. Diglipur attracts tourists both domestic and foreign in plenty because of its unique feature, Natural Beauty, Saddle Peak, the highest peak of the Andaman and Nicobar Islands. Tourists come to Port Blair first and they have to reach Mayabunder via Rangat. From there they have to go to Kalighat- a village by boat by crossing a small creek and from there they reach Diglipur by Bus. Otherwise, one can directly go to Diglipur from Port Blair by boat. But now Andaman and Nicobar Administration has successfully constructed a bus route directly from Port Blair to Diglipur and thereby one can go to Diglipur by road transport also. However they will have to cross some small creeks by the vehicle ferry.

Trade and Diglipur

The economy of the Diglipur Islands in general, consists of Trade, Commerce, Forest, Plantation, Agriculture and Tourism. The commerce of this island is divided into 5 categories namely Finance, Transport, Insurance, Store house and Advertisement. The island is connected by the ferry services and inter-island shipping services. As far as the status of the economy of this island is concerned, it is backward and is cut-off from the main stream of National Life. Due to the lack of education and less education on the part of the entrepreneurs in the field of proper exploitation of the resources, all the essential goods, industrial goods, construction goods etc. are brought from the mainland of India. The customers and consumers do not have their choice of goods. They are often compelled to buy the goods, which are sold by the traders who bring goods from the traders of Mainland and Port Blair . Though a lot of goods and services can be produced and manufactured in this island itself, they are brought from the Mainland of India and Port Blair.

As far as the trading activity is concerned, the Diglipur Islands is one of the excellent growing trading centres. Number of wholesale provision shops, retail shops, number of commercial establishments, number of schools, institutions, hotels, tourists spots, vegetable stalls have been increasing. Cultivators sell their products to the wholesale agents who come from different islands of this territory. Hence it is an important place of interest attracting everyone. By taking the production in terms of quantity of the paddy and other cultivation, Diglipur Island has been defined as "Granary of Andaman and Nicobar Islands" by the researcher Dr. N. Rajavel in 1990.

Trade Entrepreneurs

Entrepreneurs are the kingpins of the business not merely men willing to trade for a profit but who are able to exploit the available resources in the right manner, at the right time, and in the process of creation of more goods and employment, and thereby offer a better standard of living to the people of the region. In fact the total population of these islands depend fully on the trade entrepreneurs of this island. It is not exaggeration to say that the entrepreneurs do business ventures because doing business in Diglipur Island, a far away place from the mainland is not as easy as a normal man can think. In the present work of study on the workings of entrepreneurs is confined only to the entrepreneurs from Trade Sector. The questionnaires have been served only to the trade units. Hence, entrepreneurs in this paper mean only trade entrepreneurs of the Diglipur Island.

Methodology

To study the working of traders, a semi-structured questionnaire has been constructed. The questionnaires have been served on a sample of 80 trade entrepreneurs selected for the purpose of this study on random basis. Questions on general working of the trade entrepreneurs were asked. Of the total sample, 13 questionnaires were incomplete and 10 traders did not submit the questionnaires. Hence, only 67 questionnaires have been taken for the analysation purpose. Besides the questionnaires, an informal interview was also held to know their present problem and to know their valuable suggestions. A brief account of the questionnaires is given in Table 1. The results of the analysation and interpretation are presented.

Table 1

Account for Questionnaires

Sl. No.	*Particulars*	*Number*
01	Total Questionnaires Distributed	80
02	Total Questionnaires Received back	70
03	Questionnaires Incomplete	03
04	Net Questionnaires taken for Study	67

Analysation

Based on the particulars submitted by the respondent traders of and collected from the Diglipur Island, the data are analysed, interpreted and presented to the learned readers and users of this study. The workings of the traders are analysed under the following heads.

1. Classification
2. Educational Qualifications
3. Nature Of Business
4. Number of Employees
5. Capital Investment
6. Place of Purchase
7. Place of Sales
8. Operational Particulars
9. Problems

Classification

The traders in Diglipur are classified of the basis of forms of business organizations. As far as the trade units are concerned, the nature of business is same in almost all the cases. As a first analysation, it is found that the ownership of the trade units in Diglipur is of three types namely - Sole proprietorship, Partnership firms, Co- operatives. The number of trade units under the each form of organization is given in table – 2. The table clearly pictures that the more number of units are in the form of sole proprietorship, which is followed, by the form of 89.6% are sole proprietorship forms, 5 representing 7.5% units are partnership form and only two units representing 2.9% are co-operative forms. No company form of Trade Unit is found in the Diglipur Island.

Table 2
Form of Business Organization

Sl. No.	*Forms*	*No. of units*	*Percentage*
1	Sole trader/Proprietorship	60	89.6%
2.	Partnership	05	7.5%
3.	Co – operatives	02	2.9%
4.	Others	-	-
	Total	67	100

Source: Primary Data - 2003

Educational Qualifications

The education plays a vital roe in the development of Entrepreneurship in the entrepreneur. The educational qualification of the owner, manager or the managing director as the case may have been taken for the purpose of this analysation. This is because, they only manage the unit and they only take the decision in the unit. On the basis of the data collection, the educational qualification are classified as Below metric, Metric , Graduation, Post Graduation, and Others. Table 3 shows the number

Table 3
Educational Qualifications of Traders

Sl. No.	*Educational Qualifications*	*No.of Respondents*	*Percentage*
1.	Metric and above	55	82
2.	Graduation	09	13.4
3.	Post Graduation	02	1.5
4.	Others	02	3.0
	Total	67	100.0

Source: Primary Data - 2003

of entrepreneurs with their educational qualifications. It reveals that majority of the respondents are qualified as metric and below metric. Of the total respondents, 55 responding 82% are metric and below metric. Only nine, 13.4% are graduates and one trader, 10% is post graduate degree holders.

Nature of Business

It includes Wholesale trade and /or Retail trade. The workings of the traders greatly depend upon the nature of their business. In Diglipur, sixteen traders representing 23.9% are doing only wholesale business and fifty-eight traders representing 86.6% are doing wholesale as well as retail trade. Table 4 gives the particulars about the nature of the business. It is understood from the interviews that the traders from nearby villages of the Diglipur Town purchase from the traders of the Diglipur Bazaar Area. So all the wholesale traders establish their business near the jetty/harbour.

Table 4

Nature of Business

Sl. No.	*Nature of Business*	*No. of units*	*Percentage*
1	Whole sale alone	09	13.4
2.	Retail alone	--	--
3.	Retail and wholesale	58	86.6
4.	Others	--	--
	Total	67	100.0

Source: Primary Data – 2003

Nature of Employees

Another important factor that determines the work efficiency of the traders is the number of employees appointed and their workings. The traders of the Diglipur Island appoint their labourers ranging form 01 to 05 nos. this is clearly shown in table 5. The table shows that the majority of

Table 5

Number of Employees Appointed by the Traders

Sl. No.	*No. of Employees*	*No. of units*	*Percentage*
1	01	05	7.4
2.	02	42	62.7
3.	03	05	7.4
4.	04	09	13.5

Sl. No.	No. of Employees	No. of units	Percentage
4.	04	09	13.5
5	05 and above	06	9.0
	Total	67	100.0

Source: Primary Data - 2003

the traders appoint 02 employees/labourers. Sixty-seven traders representing 62.7% appointed only two employees and six trade units representing 9.0% appointed upto five employees. The main reason for this is that they have to maintain unnecessary books and ledgers for the employees and they answerable to the labour rules.

Capital Investment

Finance is lifeblood of the business. Capital investment is the main spring of any unit. The capital investment by the Diglipur Traders in their trade units is classified into six heads as follows because all traders in this island came under the small business.

1. Upto Rs. 1,00,000
2. From Rs. 1,00,000 to Rs. 2,00,000
3. From Rs. 2,00,000 to Rs. 3,00,000
4. From Rs. 3,00,000 to Rs. 4,00,000
5. From Rs. 4,00,000 to Rs. 5,00,000
6. Rs. 5,00,000 an above.

Table 6

Capital Investment of Traders

Sl. No.	Capital Investment	No. of units	Percentage
1	Below 1,00,000	33	49.2
2.	1,00,000 to 2,00,000	15	22.4
3.	2,00,000 to 3,00,000	10	14.9
4.	3,00,000 to 4,00,000	05	07.5
5	4,00,000 to 5.00,000	02	03.0
6	5,00,000 and Above	02	03.0
	Total	67	100.0

Source: Primary Data - 2003

Table 6 shows the Capital Investment Classifications of the Traders. The table shows that the maximum number of traders working with the total capital investment of below Rs. 2,00,000. Thirty-three representing 49.2% are working with the total capital investment of Rs. 1,00,000 and below. One representing 22.4% of respondents are with capital investment of Rs. 2,00,000. Only two trade units representing 3% are with a capital investment of more than Rs. 5,00,000.

Place of Purchase

Though the buying and selling activities are the functions of traders, the purchase is the actual primary activity of any trader. Here, purchase means the purchase of goods for the purpose of sale. If any trader spends more amounts towards the purchase of goods besides the cost of goods, then no doubt, he will certainly have to wed with loss. So, place of purchase has become very important, particularly places like Diglipur Island. The traders of Diglipur Island occupy a special position like a doctor among the patients. Wherever be the place, the trader of this island must take steps to procure the goods and they must bring to the Diglipur Island. Otherwise, the public will face a lot of problems.

Table 7

Place of Purchase

Sl. No.	*Place of Purchase*	*No. of units*	*Percentage*
1	From Mainland	03	04.5
2.	From Port Blair	35	50.2
3.	From Other Islands	17	25.4
4.	Locally	12	17.9
	Total	67	100.0

Source: Primary Data - 2003

Table 7 shows the place of purchase. It is classified form the data collected as Locally, From other islands, and From Port Blair. As per the table, 35 traders representing sharing 52.2% purchases from Port Blair, the only city in the union territory of Andaman & Nicobar Islands. This group includes the wholesale traders. 12 traders purchase from local whole sellers and 17 traders representing 25.4% purchase from the islands. Three traders representing 4.5% of the total respondent traders procure directly from the Mainland of India.

Place of Sales

Sales is the major source of finance. It is the revenue provider. Sales is one of the ways to facilitate the consumers to buy the goods and services. On the basis of the data collected, the place of sales by the

Diglipur traders is grouped as Locally, To other islands and To Port Blair. Table 08 gives the particulars about the places of Sales by the Traders of Diglipur island. 63 traders representing 94.0% sell goods locally. It includes both retailers and whole sellers. Three out of 67 sharing 4.5% told that they have been selling in both locally and to the traders of Port Blair. One expressed that he sells goods to other island traders.

Table 8
Place of Sales

Sl. No.	*Place of Sales*	*No. of units*	*Percentage*
1	To Port Blair	03	04.5
2.	To Other Islands	01	01.5
3.	Locally	63	94.0
	Total	67	100.0

Source: Primary Data - 2003

Operational Particulars

Computers, Vehicles, Services of the Consultants, Agencies etc., have become very important like the booster dose for a growing child. Depending upon the size of the trade unit, the traders may go for additional operational aids such as computers, vehicles, services of agent, clustered goods, service of chartered accountant etc. Table 9 shows the operating particulars about the traders of Diglipur Island. One surprising point to be noted is that 19 traders 28.4% have appointed agents to sell goods. It shows that these traders have high volume of sales. Fifty-three traders have expressed that they maintain accounts and 34 respondents pay income tax. Twenty-four respondents have vehicles of two wheelers and four wheelers. As far as the competition is concerned, almost all have the problem of competition from each other.

Table 9
Particulars about Operational Information

Sl. No.	*Operational Information*	*No. of units*	*Percentage*
1	Vehicles	24	35.8
2.	Service from Agencies	19	28.4
3.	Maintaining Accounts	53	79.0
4.	Paying Income Tax	34	50.7
5	Competitors	49	73.1
6	Selling Vegetables also	03	04.5
7	Using Computers	19	28.4

Source: Primary Data - 2003

Problems

The problems are the speed breakers of the growing units. No creature in the world is without problems. Everyone faces problem. The traders of Diglipur are not exception to this. They face many problems like financial problems, transport problems, labour problems, power problems. Table 10 shows the problems faced by the traders of Diglipur. 49 respondents have expressed that they face more problems in finance. They said that their business would have been increased if they have enough finance with them. 29 respondents stated that they face transport problem. 08 told that they could not get power and had to overcome this major problem. Few traders have their own generators. 67 sadly expressed that they are suffering much due to the power problem.

Table 10

Problems Facing the Traders

Sl. No.	*Problems*	*No. of units*	*Percentage*
1	Finance	41	61.2
2.	Transport	29	43.3
3.	Labour	08	11.9
4.	Power	06	09.0
	Others	11	16.4

Source: Primary Data - 2003

Findings

Trade in Andaman & Nicobar Islands has been considered as "the life giving aspect" to the people of this territory and so the case of Diglipur Island. The local administration and government of India has been encouraging both the industry and trade. Diglipur is named as " Granary of Andaman & Nicobar Islands" (Rajavel 990). It is a resourceful island. Traders in this island are developing. 89.6% of the units are sole proprietorship form of business organization. 7.5% of the units are partnership form of organization. 82% of the total traders are qualified only below Metric and Metric. 13.4% are graduates.

Majority of the traders is doing retail business. 86.6% are doing retail business and 13.4% are doing both wholesale and retail business. Majority of the traders appointed is only two employees. Such traders constitute 62.7%. As far as the capital investment is concerned, majority of the traders has their capital investment upto Rs. 1,00,000. Only very limited traders of the sample have invested more than 5,00,000 as their capital. 59.7% of the sample expressed that they buy goods from Port Blair. 25.4% expressed as they buy from nearby islands but 17.9%of the traders purchase goods locally. Majority of the sample traders (94.4%) sells goods locally and 4.5% traders sell goods both locally and to Port Blair.

In Diglipur, 79.1% traders maintain account and 50.7% traders pay income tax. These traders have high volume of sales/business and 35.8% of the traders have vehicles of two wheelers/four wheelers. The traders in Diglipur are not free from problems. Though they face a lot of problems, 61.2% of the traders told that they financial problems, 43.3% traders face transport problems, 11.9% face labour problems and 9.0% of the sample traders told that they face power problems.

Suggestions

The following suggestions are offered for the overall development of the trading business and to overcome the problems of traders in the islands of Diglipur.

1. A separate Trade Development Department is to be setup in these islands. Those who have done the research work on the trade are to be recruited and appointed with the Authority and Responsibilities. The conventional method of making some officer as in-charge of the proposed department will not bring the expected result.
2. A regular cargo boat to and from Diglipur is to be operated every day from Port Blair. The boat has to touch only Mayabunder. One more boat touching all the other islands with a full single day round trip is suggested.
3. Trade finance scheme is to be introduced with the subsidies and bounties.
4. A cold storage and a warehouse are to be constructed in Diglipur.
5. To drive away the power problem, one more Generator set is to be established in this island.
6. To encourage the trading activity and industrial activities, the local government should take steps to bring awareness about the available resources in this island , method of exploiting the resources, how to approach officers of the different categories, available facilities, concessions, subsidies etc., For this purpose the local administration may take all the steps to advertise the necessary information useful to the traders. It may make use of the All India Radio Station for the advertisements etc.

7. The traders of Diglipur Island are to be given training on how to start the new ventures, how to maintain the accounts, letter writing, marketing technical aspects, and quality training in the field of Accounts, book keeping, Business laws, Management and Technique of facing challenges etc.

Conclusion

Once the impediments in the path of the Trade Development in the Bay Islands particularly in the Diglipur Island are removed, and a training is given to all the traders of the Diglipur Island, a Cold Storage & a Warehouse are constructed in the Diglipur Islands and an effective strategy is formulated in the light of the suggestions given, and if the same is implemented carefully through the dedicated and qualified officers without the yes masters, butter-men, and with out the interference of the political and other unwanted factors and with full meaningful principles, the workings of these traders will get merit rating an will increase the standard of living of the people of this island which will push the economy of the Andaman & Nicobar Islands which will contribute a lot to the over all economic development of India.

19

Management of Traffic Jam

Introduction

India is still considered as a developing country and so the case of Andaman and Nicobar Islands. This is due to many reasons such as increasing population, low per capita real income, poor Infrastructural facilities, under utilisation of resources, barriers in the labour mobilization, Mass poverty, high cost of living, absolute methods of production, lack of skilled personnel, lack of entrepreneurial talent, non-economic factors like favoritism, nepotism and corruption etc. economic development requires efficient, dedicated and clean administration and management at all levels. The political, cultural and social developments have no meaning without the economic development and prosperity. This paper is restricted to only our Green Paradise, picturesque, enchanting beautiful and resourceful A & N Islands with special reference to the Management of Traffic Jam.

A & N Islands

A & N Islands, situated in the Bay of Bengal are surrounded by Burma, Thailand, Malaysia and Indonesia. The islands constitute the most isolated part of India Union, stretching in North South Direction, separated from the Mainland of India vast stretches of sea. The Andaman groups of islands are separated from Nicobar Group of Islands by 10-degree channel. This territory, comprising an area of 8293 square kilometers in a group of picturesque islands. Port Blair, the capital of this Bay Islands is connected with the Mainland by both sea and air routes. The seat of Administration is situated in Port Blair City.

Economic Status

Only from the recent past, these Islands witness some development, which can be counted for economic development. Number of industrial units, trade units, commercial units, travel units started increasing by showing a growing trend at a lower rate. The Chamber of Commerce and Industry, Associations of Small Scale Units, The Department of Commerce in JNRM and Trade Associations have been contributing their possible efforts to the growth of these islands.

Role of Transport

Transport plays a vital role in the economic development of Andaman and Nicobar Islands because the quick transports help in opening up remote and inaccessible regions, promotes labour mobility, protects the market, helps in the movement of raw materials, fuels, machinery, finished goods, promote industries and widening the people's out look which is very important factor. For accelerating the economic growth particularly in A & N Islands, it is not merely the physical resources which are required but also progressive out look of the people indicating urge for economic uplift and ready responsiveness to new suggestions. In fact, the modern out look of the people is important determinant of economic growth.

Warning

Though this green territory has a lot of potential resources, number of problems and challenges face these islands. Increasing unemployment problem, decreasing productivity, increasing inefficiency, decreasing in work culture and increasing uncontrollable population, dislocation of monsoons are some of the problems facing these resourceful islands.

Now, another serious problem facing these islands and which has been growing rapidly and is going to be the biggest obstacle, impediments of the economic growth of these islands is the growing number of transports. The author warns i.e social warning that the Andaman and Nicobar Islands will find it very difficult to provide space for parking the vehicles shortly if the administration does not take proper steps to check it. Every office, school, colleges, secretariat, and all the other organisations, the city roadside area, water sports complex, harbours, airports, bus terminus, beaches, science centre, temples, mosque, churches, vegetable markets and other places will have acute shortage of space for parking the vehicle. Such problem will be resulting in terrific traffic jam, accidents, delay in travel and in tension travel.

Traffic Jam — Present Scenario

From Monday to Saturday, the roads are full of transports of different varieties. The traffic gets thickly concentrated everyday from 0800 hours (8.00AM) onwards and that such concentration goes and prevails upto 2000 hours (8.00PM). But during some important days, the thick transport concentration goes even beyond 2000 hours (8.00PM).. The acute traffic jam takes place everyday between 0800 hours (8.00AM) and 0900 hours (9.00AM) hours, between 1200 hours (12.00Noon) and 1300 hours (1.00PM) and between 1400 hours (2.00 PM) and 1530 hours (3.30 PM)in almost all the places particularly in front of all the schools.

The school children move here and there very fast to catch their vehicles, buses to their home and finally they met with accidents. The traffic jam creates severe noise pollution, air pollution besides the accidents and irritating travel. Vehicles could not go freely. Sometimes the traffic jam stops the emergency cases going to hospital and thereby the emergency case has to forget this world for ever. Even one fears to walk on the roadside. The author has carefully verified the extent of traffic jam. It is extremly more only at the time of the School timings i.e from 0800 hours (8.00AM) to 0900 hours (9.00AM) hours, from 1200 hours (12.00Noon) to 1300 hours (1.00PM) and from 1400 hours (2.00 PM) to 1530 hours (3.30 PM). This situation prevails not only in the Capital City but also in almost all the places where the schools are functioning. The important traffic jam places are in front of Vivekananda School, Model School, Boys School Middle Point, Nirmala School, Carmel School, KV I School, Ummath School, Head Post Office, RTO Office, Telephone Bhavan, Ghandhi Market, Mohanpura School, Mohanpura Market, Rathinam Market, Delanipur Market etc., Moreover during the visit of any VIP, the public faces painful problem due to the long traffic jam. Really the traffic jam is a heavy headache to the public and to the Andaman and Nicobar Administration.

Management of Traffic Jam

To remove the traffic jam is absolutely impossible in the present scenario and situation. But it can be managed to reduce the concentration of the traffic jam. A proper Planning, effective Organising, dedicated Staffing, clear-cut Communication, impartial Control and sincere Coordination on the part of the authorities will certainly reduce the Traffic Jam. By analysing the present situation, warning, increasing population of vehicles, importance of education, need of the happy life, possibilities on the part of the departments and the schools etc., few measures are given in the name of suggestions. The learned Persons, Officers, Principals and respected Teachers and the Critics of this articles are requested to go through this writings and are further requested to cooperate to reduce the traffic jam if they consider the suggestions are good. Their comments are also invited.

1. The drivers of the commercial vehicles - lorries, trucks, auto-rickshaws, taxies, carriers etc., are to be given orientation about the

traffic rules. It is estimated that about 80% of the drivers do not completely know about the traffic rules. If possible, they are to be called batch by batch and they should be given extensive training for a period of atleast 10 days. As far as the cost of conducting the training programme, both the administration and the drivers/vehicle owners should bear in the ratio of 60% : 40%. The government/ administration alone cannot bear the full expenses.

2. At the end of the training period, each driver is to be given a Driving Training Completion Certificate/Card (DTCC) and the drivers are expected to carry the Card always with them. The drivers who do not take the training should not be allowed to drive at all. The action should be taken by the Police Department.

3. If the administration desires, the author will prepare a model of orientation training programme including the cost aspects, steps to start the programme and coordinate the programme initially for some time.

4. The main shopping areas like Aberdeen Bazaar, Junglighat, Dhilanipur, Rangat Main Bazaar Area, Diglipur Main Bazaar Area etc., should me made free from the parking of vehicles in front of the shops, hotels and the commercial establishments. The starting points of the Shopping Area from the different directions are to be fixed and no vehicle is permitted to be parked in side the Shopping Area Only the going vehicles are to be allowed to pass the area without any stoppage and without horn. A proper provision for parking the vehicle of different types is to be made on the side of the road in Just 100 meters before the starting point of the Shopping Areas. It can be done easily at the present structure.

5. For example, Junglighat is a Shopping Area. The starting points are the Radha Govindhan Temple from the North Direction, Old CCS unit/ Transport Corporation Building from the South Direction, Junglighat Jetty from the West Direction are the starting points. Parking the vehicles must be prohibited in between these points. Then, road side area available in front of the Radha Govindhan Temple is to be used for the parking the vehicles both four wheelers and two wheelers. The concerned authorities must make the parking lines for the two and four wheelers on the road. People let them walk after parking the vehicles for shopping since it is good for health and will reduce the sugar and BP problems However going vehicles are to be allowed without any stop and horn in side the Shopping Area. The

same manner, the road side area just next to the Transport Corporation of India Building, and road side area available opposite to Vijay Bhag are to be used for parking the vehicles. As far as the Junglighat Jetty Starting Point is concerned, at present all commercial trucks are parked on the road though there is enough space for parking in the place meant for. May be one reason or other, they park their vehicles on the road. They may be advised to park in side the parking maidan. Arrangements are to be made to have two gates for going inside and coming outside in two extremes for the commercial vehicles particularly the trucks as "IN" and "OUT". In between these points good number of light vehicles can be parked. Like wise, a systematic plan is to be made and the same may be carefully implemented.

6. As far as the Aberdeen Bazaar is concerned, the starting point may me Model School from one direction. From the State Library gate to YMCA shopping complex, the road side area can be used for parking. This is also an example for the consideration. What I meant to say is that the vehicles are to be parked only in the areas identified and earmarked for the parking. In the parking areas the speed of the vehicles are to be just 30 Kms only.

7. The Traffic Islands are to be provided with high level traffic umbrella with lighting facilities. The signal given by the Traffic Island Police is to be clearly visible to the drivers. He should be given reflecting plates for the " STOP" in Red Colour and "GO" in Green Colour.

8. The heavy vehicles lorries and trucks etc., are to be are to be diverted during the school timings. The VIP Road, RGT Road, Phonies Bay Road may be used for such diversion after the careful study.

9. Another serious problem is the traffic jam in front of the Schools both at the time of starting and closing hours i.e from 0800 hours (8.00AM) to 0900 hours (9.00AM) hours, from 1200 hours (12.00Noon) to 1300 hours (1.00PM) and from 1400 hours (2.00 PM) to 1530 hours (3.30 PM). This situation prevails not only in the Capital City but also in also in almost all the places where the schools are functioning. All vehicles are taken and dumped in front of the schools just one hour before the closing hours. Other vehicles have to stand in Q which runs more than one kilometer length making the full area as traffic jam with noise pollution and air pollution. This sometimes resulted in heavy accidents between the vehicles and thereby they make further traffic jam. So it is suggested to have a small adjustment in every school. The responsibilities are completely with not only the Principal and also with every teacher of the school.

10. Now almost all the schools start by 9.00 AM and closes by 3.00PM. The first suggestion is that the Principals may meet at one place and discuss this issue and they can have two types of timings. That is some schools may have their School timings as from 9.00AM to 3.00PM and some schools may have their school timings as from 10.00AM to 4.00PM. The author believes that the traffic jam in general will be reduced to some extent.

11. Again all the schools have the prayer system which is very very important. Normally all the students are compelled to participate in the prayer. But one thing everybody must notice that no college is adopting the prayer system. No one knows the real reason. In every higher secondary school, the higher classes are the 10th Standard, 11th Standard and 12th Standard. They are little bit matured also. So they may be exempt in participating in the Prayer for 5 days i.e from Monday to Friday. On Saturdays the students from KG I, KGII and Class I may be given full Holiday and on Saturdays the Prayer may be made compulsory for all the classes from class II including higher classes i.e 10th –12th Standard.

12. The class hours for the students of 10th – 12th Standard for the first five days i.e from Monday to Friday may be from 10.00 AM to 4.00 PM and on the Saturday the class timings may be from 9.00 AM to 3.00 PM because they have to attend the prayer. So the vehicles which carry the students of higher classes will come one hour after the other vehicles both in the mornings and evenings. On Saturdays normally the number of vehicles will be less due to the holiday for the KGI, KGII and I Standard. For the first five days students from the IX Standard will assist the teachers and principal in the prayer.

13. From Monday to Friday class leaving timings may be like this
    (a) Nursery, KG I & KG II 12.00 Noon
    (b) I to IV Standard 2.00 PM
    (c) V to IX Standard 2.45 PM
    (d) X to XII Standard 3.30 PM

    For Saturday the class leaving timings may be:

    (a) II to IV Standard 2.00 PM
    (b) V to IX Standard 2.45 PM.
    (c) X to XII Standard 3.00 PM

    By doing so the movements of vehicles will be very less and there won't be any traffic jam in front of the schools. The Principals must instruct the students to tell and inform the parents to come only in time to pickup them. No vehicle should come in advance and park in front of the school before the timings. Moreover, the preparation of the timetable for the students will become easy by allocating the works to the teachers at optimum level. Planning and Organising, Communication, Controlling and Coordination will be very easy and logical if the above timings are adopted.

14. Sometimes, the Principals may be interested to have the Prayers with all the students of the school and they don't want to call the senior students by 10.00AM. In that case, alternatively, they can compel the students to inform their parents to drop them well in time. That is, those students who come by four wheelers they have to come at or before 8.00AM and the other two wheelers may come after 8.00AM but before 830AM. Of course, this arrangements will certainly reduce the traffic jam to certain extent. The Principal, Carmel School has started adopting this arrangement as a test checking. Even in that case also, four where traffic jam and two wheeler traffic jam may arise in the long run. Even in this arrangement also, the schools must adopt the system of leaving timings as suggested above with slight modification. This is because all the students come to school by 9.00AM. The Principals who wish to adopt this model suggestion may have the following leaving timings to reduce the Traffic Jam. Here all the students will attend the Prayer.

    (a) Nursery, KG I & KG II 12.00 Noon
    (b) I to IV Standard 2.00 PM
    (c) V to IX Standard 2.45 PM
    (d) X to XII Standard 3.00 PM

15. For all National Festivals and School Celebrations, only the students from V Standard to IX standard may be called to participate and students from X Standard to XII Standard may be asked to organise the functions. Each function must have the maximum duration of 60 – 90 minutes. The participating students will be asked to leave the school first and after 30 minutes only the organising students may be allowed to leave the school. By doing so the traffic jam will be reduced considerably.

16. Now the government owned STS bus service seems to be less visible. It requires a thorough study and the whole department is to be overhauled through a systematic examination and a meaningful research. It is possible and it can be done. The department and the system may be rejuvenated and revitalized. The buses can be operated under the ownership of the government. By doing so, the buses can

be procured and they may be operated as school trips besides the normal scheduled route. In that case also, the traffic jam in front of the schools may be reduced considerably.

17. The Private people may be called to operate buses for the schools in a very disciplined way. Here the instructions are to be prepared and to be given to the owners of the buses by fixing responsibilities. But the feasibility is to be checked carefully.

Conclusion

Different types of alternative models have been given above to check the traffic jam. Whatever is applicable to the system of school, the principals may practice it first on the test checking basis. If they find easy and don't feel any problem, they are requested to adopt the system to reduce the traffic jam. It will be a great social responsibility on the part of the schools. Giving suggestion is very easy. But it is very difficult to Practice it. Only at the time of implementation and execution of the suggested ideas, different types of problems and objections may arise. The parents whose two or three children are studying in the same school in different classes have to come in different timings to pickup them. Really it is very difficult on the part of such parents. But if the children are waiting for a while in the school itself till the higher-class brother or sister comes, then there will be no problem. Here it is the question of a light adjustment. However, the above measures are suggested only after the careful analysis by taking the welfare of the schools, students and society at large and as a whole. Of course, initially, no doubt, there will be really problems to implement the new suggestions as generally people resist for change. But in due course, they themselves will realise and do practice and will extent their cooperation. The whole suggestions are to be carefully analysed with the learned persons by taking the present problems facing the islands and the author's warning and the economic conditions of this green islands. Since it is related to the traffic jam, the whole exercise is to be coordinated by the Police Department. The Principals of the schools are requested to prepare the manual of instruction in the light of the above suggestions if they considers these measures are practically possible. One should not think that it is the duty of only the Police Department and Principals of Educational Institutions to take the responsibility of reducing the traffic jam. The parents and the public also have the equal responsibility in the matter of reducing traffic jam. Everybody should full heartedly cooperate to reduce the traffic jam and to make this Green Islands as Green Paradise with Secured, Standard and Pollution Free Life.

20

Role of Tourism in Economic Changes in Bay Islands

Abstract

The Economy of the Andaman & Nicobar Islands consists of the Three Major Sectors namely Agriculture, Business, and Marine. The Business Sector in Andaman & Nicobar Islands is further divided in to Industry, Commerce and Trade sectors. Tourism is a branch of Industrial sector. This article concentrates on the changes (its growth) in the tourism industry in Andaman & Nicobar Islands since independence, and how the tourism industry brought change in the other socio-economic factors like education, employment, savings, industrial units, shops and commercial establishments by bringing a huge change itself. It is proved through the correlation analysis. The only sector upon the whole territory depends at present is the Business sector. Even in Business sector, commerce and trade have been recording positive changes in growing trend. Tourism Industry is at present in infant stage and this is the only hope of this territory for its economic development. It has recorded a marvelous growth in terms of arrival tourists. The numbers of tourists (foreign and domestic) come to these islands since independence has been increasing. The increase in number of tourists both foreign and domestic for the year 1980 was 139.9% over the year 1970; for the 1990 it is 251.4% over the year 1980 and it is 218.3% in 2000 over 1990. But taking the year 1970 as the base year, the increase in number of tourists has recorded a growth of 139.9% in 1980; 742.9% in 1990 and a marvelous growth rate of 2582.8% in the year 2000. The correlation analysis shows that there a constructive positive correlation between the tourism industry and the other elements and factors by recording its potentiality in these Green Paradise. Necessary arrangements are to be made to attract more number of tourists on the economic ground. Suitable suggestions are offered to strengthen this economic activity of tourism in this Green Solid Paradise on the Blue Liquid Surface.

What is Socio-Economic Change?

Many authors have tried their level best to define the Socio-economic change. But those definitions were not fully inclusive. Since it is a very vast area with vast scope it is very difficult to define fully. So here in this paper, though it is not covering all areas, a simple definition is given. The term Socio-Economic changes is defined as a process in which discernible significant alternation in the structure and functioning of a particular Socio -economic system. Significant change in social behaviour, social structure and cultural values, education, employment, capital mobilization, habit of savings of the people, number of educational institutions, number of shops and commercial establishments, industrial units etc. This is called Socio-economic Change.

Andaman & Nicobar Islands Since Independence

Andaman and Nicobar Islands, by virtue of its strategic geographical location in the Bay of Bengal and rich Natural Resources, attracts and receives great attention. The Bay Islands, as it is also known, constitute the remotest region of our country. The inky, blue waters of the Bay of Bengal and the Andaman Sea, once coined as KALAPANI (the Black water) indicating the dreaded transportation, punishment of the British Government of India and the overwhelming grandeur of vast, cloud ridden skies make them a domain of unsullied nature. "KALAPANI" is all that many have heard of a term that for centuries conjured up the dark vision of forbidden land surrounded by vast sheets of deep water, unapproachable and hostile. The inhabitants of these islands are scattered far flung and wide over a distance of 720 kms. Some of them are found established well in a few towns and innumerable small villages. But due to the location of these small villages, inhabitants are cut-off from civilization and from the source of supply of essential commodities. The towns and small villages have started flourishing only recently, because of the harbour facilities that have been provided in these islands and slow progress of shipping and other transport facilities. Andaman and Nicobar islands is a green paradise which stretches its long arm of welcome to the mainland across the sea, an outpost pulsating some pioneering activities.

The population of Andaman & Nicobar Islands when we gained Independence was just 30,000 of which the tribal population was about 12,000. Since Independence, the population started increase, people from the mainland started finding these islands suitable for living, Administration also invited people from mainland for the settlement, Jobs were vacant in every field, possibilities of setting the industrial units have become visible, academicians, anthropologists, economists, researchers identified the resources etc. These great changes have now induced the social scientists, anthropologists to be engaged in the study of the social and economic change.

Factors Responsible for Change

There are many factors responsible for Socio-economic changes of Andaman & Nicobar Islands. Such factors are identified. They are Demographic Factor, Technological Factor, Cultural Factor, Revolution Factor, War Factor, Legislation Factor, Planning Factor, Education Factor, Trade Factor, Commerce Factor, Industrial Factor, and Tourism Factor. Actually, the changes are the result of the effective role of one or more of these factors on the Socio-economic surface of the particular region or country or area. Actually all factors are to be taken to study the contribution made by them for the Socio-economic changes of Andaman & Nicobar Islands. As you all know it is very difficult to present a paper by taking all factors in seminar due to the time factor i.e want of time, as far as this paper is concerned, Tourism Factor is being taken for the presentation. The main reason for taking Tourism for presentation is that this is the factor which has close relation with the society contributing to the economic growth. There is no doubt that A & N Islands is a Tourist's paradise. The Natural Scenic Beauty, serpentine creeks, palm fringed sandy beaches, corals and unpolluted environment are great attractions for the tourists - both domestic and foreign.

Tourism in A & N Islands

Tourism is really the next change in the diary of Andaman & Nicobar Islands. The union territory of A&N Islands realised the importance of tourism in this Nature's Gifted Paradise. Efforts were made to declare this economic activity as industry and as a result, as well as with a view to develop the tourism in the union territory of Andaman & Nicobar Islands, the then Lt. Governor (Administrator) of A & N Islands had been pleased to order that 'Tourism' will be treated as an industry in A & N Islands. This has been enabling those, engaged in tourism, promotional activities in the whole of the union territory of A & N Islands to become eligible for concessions/incentives as applicable to the economic industrial sector from time to time where ever such schemes are relevant to tourism activities. Concessions are also given to and made available to classified hotels, restaurants, purchase of luxury cars, coaches, boats etc by tour operators, construction of amusement parks, recreation centers, auditorium, handicrafts emporiums, rope ways, institutions teaching surfing, skiing, trekking etc.

Changes in Tourism

Enough data were not available to analyse the change of tourism since independence. However, with the great difficulties and from the reliable sources, the data could be collected from the year 1970 onwards. Even then, for few years, the data were not fully available. So the analysation has been done only with the help of the available data. To highlight the changes took place in the Tourism Factor and with a view to have a bird's eye view on the growth of tourism, the total number of tourists arrived in the Andaman & Nicobar Islands is given in the table 1.

Table 1

Total Number of Tourists Arrived Into A & N Islands

Year	*Total Number of Tourists*	*% increase over the Previous Year*
1970	1100	–
1975	2000	81.8
1978	4000	100.0
1979	4397	9.9
1980	9596	118.2
1981	10005	4.3
1982	14546	45.4
1983	15837	8.9
1984	19152	20.9
1985	22555	17.8
1986	22733	0.8
1987	33676	48.1
1988	38252	13.6
1989	42359	10.7
1990	33716	20.4 (–)
1991	34490	2.3

1992	38252	10.9
1993	36771	3.9(–)
1994	54535	48.3
1995	68339	25.3
2000	96049	40.5

Source: Tourism Department, A&N Administration, Port Blair, Rajavel, 1990.

It is clear from the above table that the number of tourists arrived into these islands has been increasing since 1978 onwards except in 1990. Growth in total number of tourists arrived into these islands has been increasing. Negative growth has been recorded in the year 1990 and 1993. The main reasons are frequent changes and cancellations of ship and flights. Another reason is the decrease in the number of tourists from USSR. The variation in the number of foreign tourists is also one of the reasons for the fluctuations in the growth of total tourists. . The increase in number of tourists both foreign and domestic for the year 1980 was 139.9% over the year 1970; for the 1990 it is 251.4% over the year 1980 and it is 218.3% in 2000 over 1990. But taking the year 1970 as the base year, the increase in number of tourists has recorded a growth of 139.9% in 1980; 742.9% in 1990 and a marvelous growth rate of 2582.8% in the year 2000. Declaration of Tourism as Industry in these islands by giving all benefits such as concessions, subsidies, incentives etc, by the then Lt. Governor of A&N islands during the year 1987 was the main favourable reason for the growth of tourism particularly domestic tourism. A lot of hotels, restaurants, tourism facilities, lodges, tour operators, travel agents, transport came into existence only after the declaration of tourism as industry.

Economic Changes and Tourism

As is already told that the tourism is a smokeless Industry is only hope of the economic growth of these islands. Tourism, in terms of number of units has recorded a marvelous and significant growth. While there is a severe threatening to the industrial units particularly wood based and forest based, tourism is the only hope and factor which has brought, is bringing and will bring the positive and favourable changes in the Socio economic system of this Andaman & Nicobar Islands. Shortage of capital, shortage of entrepreneur, shortages of entrepreneurial ability, shortage of skills, shortage of technical know- how, inadequacy of transport, inadequate credit system were the situation of Andaman & Nicobar Islands.

However, for the purpose of colonization, the people were brought form mainland and even they were given free lands and other facilities for other developmental purpose. Inefficient and corrupt officers were the major political factor, which threatened the economic development of Andaman & Nicobar Islands.

But now, the whole scenario started changing. Socio-economic changes have started their visibilities in the following areas due to the growth of tourism industry in Andaman & Nicobar Islands.

1. Number of educational institutions
2. Number of industrial units
3. Number of commercial units
4. Employment
5. Per capita income
6. Small savings

Though there are many numbers of elements in the Socio economic system of our Bay islands, the following elements are taken for this present paper to examine the changes due to tourism. Data has been collected and with the help of statistical tool called correlation analysis, the relationship has been examined.

1. Education
2. Savings
3. Trade and Commerce
4. Industries and
5. Employment

Education and Tourism

Education plays a very vital role in the process of human resource development. Number of educational institutions namely schools, colleges, and institutions etc. has been increasing significantly. The tourism industry has a close positive correlation with the increase in number of educational institutions. What I want to say is that the education is one of the aspect of the social system and that too very important organ of the social system. For the increase of educational institutions, tourism growth is not the only the reason but that is also one of the reasons/ causes. But the growth of tourism industry compelled the administration to go for a separate course and as a result BTTM course has been started now renamed as BBA Tourism in JNRM Port Blair in the year1999 and the large number of applications are the evidence. More number of students are doing Diploma courses in Tourism, Courses for Tourist Guide etc. The following table shows the growth educational institutions due to the growth of tourism. This is shown in graph also.

Table 2
Socio-Economic Change — Education and Tourism

Sl. No.	Year	Tourists In Nos.	Change	Institutions In Nos.	Change
1	1970	1,100	--	104	--
2	1975	2,000	Positive	217	Positive
3	1980	9,596	Positive	243	Positive
4	1985	22,555	Positive	284	Positive
5	1990	33,716	Positive	321	Positive
6	1995	68,339	Positive	341	Positive
7	2000	96,049	Positive	361	Positive

Source: Compiled from the Basic Statistics, Annual Reports of A & N Administration, Rajavel, 1990.

Savings and Tourism

Savings is another important element of the social system. Savings is one of the factors determining the economic growth also. When other things remain constant, one can say that when income increases, the savings will also increase. There a lot of ways in which the income can be increased. Tourism is also one of the source of income of the people of Andaman & Nicobar Islands. Number of tourist travel agencies and their increase, increase in applications for the tourist and travel agency, increase in hotels and restaurants are the evidence for the tourism activity as one of the source of income. The statistical analysis shows the growth o tourism and the growth savings have positive correlation. The following table shows the growth of savings due to growth of tourism. This is shown in graph also.

Table 3
Socio-Economic Change — Savings and Tourism

S. No.	Year	Tourists In Nos.	Change	Savings In Lakhs	Change
1	1970	1,100	--	28	--
2	1975	2,000	Positive	72	Positive
3	1980	9,596	Positive	110	Positive
4	1985	22,555	Positive	183	Positive
5	1990	33,716	Positive	422	Positive
6	1995	68,339	Positive	735	Positive
7	2000	96,049	Positive	1337	Positive

Source: Compiled from the Basic Statistics, Annual Reports of A & N Administration, Rajavel, 1990.

Trade and Commerce and Tourism

Trade and commerce are the elements of economics and are the life giving aspects of these islands. If these elements favourably record the growth, then one can see the economic developments. Other wise the problems will be the result. The growth of trade and commerce has directly related with the growth of Tourism. It may not be true in the mainland but in these islands, it is true atleast to the extent of 70% though not 100%. Trade units, commercial establishments like different offices, restaurants, theaters etc are coming up based upon the needs and urges. Such needs and urges come due to the increasing tourism and allied activities. Again here also, the statistical analysis has recorded a positive correlation between the tourists arrival and number of trade and commercial units in Andaman & Nicobar Islands. The following table shows the growth of tourism and trade units. This is shown in graph also.

Table 4

Socio-Economic Change — Trade and Commerce and Tourism

Sl. No.	*Year*	*Tourists In Nos.*	*Change*	*Shops In Nos.*	*Change*
1	1970	1,100	–	379	–
2	1975	2,000	Positive	515	Positive
3	1980	9,596	Positive	813	Positive
4	1985	22,555	Positive	868	Positive
5	1990	33,716	Positive	965	Positive
6	1995	68,339	Positive	1,071	Positive
7	2000	96,049	Positive	1220	Positive

Source: Compiled from the Basic Statistics, Annual Reports of A & N Administration, Rajavel, 1990.

Industry and Tourism

Industries are the major determinant and the scale to measure the economic development of any region and so the case of Andaman & Nicobar Islands also. The more number of inflow of tourists and their increasing purchase and buying habits encourage the industrial entrepreneurs to set up many units. Increase in number of units means decrease in problems of the Socio- economic System because such increase will create and increase the employment opportunities, identification of new ventures, capital mobilization, labour mobilization, one unit will create opportunity for the next and new unit etc. This will have multiplier effect in the Socio-economic system. The increasing number of tourists has a positive correlation with the increase in number of industrial units. The following table shows the increase in number of tourists and industrial units. This is shown in graph also.

Table 5

Socio-Economic Change — Industries and Tourism

Sl. No.	Year	Tourists In Nos.	Change	Industrial Units In Nos.	Change
1	1970	1,100	–	46	–
2	1975	2,000	Positive	97	Positive
3	1980	9,596	Positive	156	Positive
4	1985	22,555	Positive	471	Positive
5	1990	33,716	Positive	869	Positive
6	1995	68,339	Positive	1180	Positive
7	2000	96,049	Positive	1374	Positive

Source: Compiled from the Basic Statistics, Annual Reports of A & N Administration, Rajavel, 1990.

Employment and Tourism

This is another important economic as well as social factor which will determine the quality of the society, quality of the economy and the Socio-Economic Growth of any region and country and so the case of Andaman & Nicobar Islands also. For any economy, the major problem is the unemployment problem which is the chronicle reason for all such anti-national causes activities. But the Tourism Industry reduces that burden considerably through its effective role in the Socio-economic system of Andaman & Nicobar Islands. As is already pointed out that the educational institutions, industrial units, etc. have been increasing due to the increasing economic activity of the smokeless industry-Tourism. As a result the employment in the private trade and commercial establishments besides the government employment has also shown a positive growth with positive correlation with the increase in number of tourists into these islands. The following tables shows the increase in tourists and increase in employment. This is shown in graph also.

Table 6

Socio-Economic Change — Employment and Tourism

Sl. No.	*Year*	*Tourists In Nos.*	*Change*	*Employment In Nos.*	*Change*
1	1970	1,100	–	819	–
2	1975	2,000	Positive	1178	Positive
3	1980	9,596	Positive	1985	Positive
4	1985	22,555	Positive	2410	Positive
5	1990	33,716	Positive	2569	Positive
6	1995	68,339	Positive	3985	Positive
7	2000	96,049	Positive	5248	Positive

Source: Compiled from the Basic Statistics, Annual Reports of A & N Administration, Rajavel, 1990.

Correlation Analysis

To find out the co-relations between the changes in tourism sector and the changes in the economy, correlation analysis is being undertaken. The number of tourist arrival both in foreign and domestic into these islands has been correlated with the different aspects of the economy namely, Educational Institutions, Savings, Shops i.e. Commercial Establishments, Industrial units and the Employment generated to test the influence of the Tourism Industry on the Economy. Surprisingly it gives a positive coefficient of correlation. The values of the coefficient of correlation are given below.

Economic Changes Due to Tourism Sector

Influence of Tourism Industry on the Economy

Sl. No.	*Correlation between Tourism and*	*Coefficient Value*
1.	Educational Institutions	+0.816189
2.	Small Savings	+0.984069
3.	Commercial Establishments	+0.886317
4.	Industrial Units	+0.967618
5.	Employment Generated	+0.985551

Problems

The UN has given recognition to the growing importance of tourism as a Socio-economic force. The contribution of tourism to job creation and economic development has been largely ignored or underestimated for many years. There are very few countries in the world with an Eco-tourism potential. The Eco-tourism potential provides many opportunities for both the protection of the environment and the development of tourism based on this huge natural resource. The future of these islands could be positively changed through the development of Eco-Tourism since it has become one of the most important and fast growing economic sectors.

But the Potential Industry Tourism is not free from the Problems. Inadequate needy Accommodations, Inadequate Transports (Bus, boats locally and ships and flights between mainland and islands), getting tickets, accumulation of sewage, frequent power cuts, inadequate water supply, nil provision for the public toilets, want of bus terminus even for private buses, absence of entertainment outside the Port Blair area, absence of fresh water facilities near the beaches, lack of Rope ways and lifts, absence of frequent folk dance tours, poor and costly postal services, absence of mile stones and of all absence of service with smiling face are some of the problems facing the Tourism Industry.

Suggestions

The following are some of the measures suggested for the development of Tourism Industry in Andaman & Nicobar Islands.

1. Islands Tourism Policy is to be prepared immediately with effective Planning.
2. Planning for the tourism is not an over night work and that too sensitive places like Andaman & Nicobar Islands. It can not be as well as it should not be decided only by one category of the people i.e either by the officers, or by bureaucrats alone. Hence, the experts, academicians, specialists from different fields are to be called and consulted and the planning for the tourism is to be made.
3. The Andaman & Nicobar Administration may construct single room accommodation at very cheaper rate in the important places of interest of A & N islands. The administration may think for the floating accommodations. For that purpose, the Private Sectors may be called and encouraged.
4. The hotels and restaurants who face the off-season problems may adopt and announce the multiple concession schemes like discount during off-season, meals on no profit no loss basis, more % of concession if they stay for more period, family tourist concession etc.
5. The Andaman & Nicobar Administration may introduce Island Air Service. A detailed scheme is given in tourism book Tourism in

Andaman & Nicobar Islands written by the author about the method of operation.

6. Milestones, Pillars and public toilets are to be constructed and they are to be carefully maintained. The tourists may be strictly instructed to adopt all such rules with a view to save our Socio-cultural life.
7. Reservation facilities for the shipping and flight services may be extended to all the areas in the islands and mainland.
8. Cable cars, Rope ways, Bus Terminus for the private buses, are to be constructed in the Port Blair.
9. Accommodation facilities for the tourists who wish to come to and go from Andaman & Nicobar Islands may be constructed near the horbour and the airport.

Conclusion

So in my conclusion, I would like stress that the only hope today for the Socio-economic development of Andaman and Nicobar Islands is the Tourism Industry. The contribution of tourism to job creation and economic development has been largely ignored or underestimated for many years. The Eco-tourism potential provides many opportunities for both the protection of the environment and the development of tourism based on this huge natural resource. The future of Andaman and Nicobar Islands could be positively changed through the development of Tourism Industry. If proper strategies with the tourism policy are constructed for the development of tourism in the light of the suggestions given and if they are implemented through the real, qualified and dedicated personnel, I am sure, that we can also contribute to the National Income of India.

21

Suggestions for Planning Tourism

Introduction

No doubt the population characteristics, resources, tourism attractions, tourism facilities, places of interest and their features, social, cultural, religious and economic aspects, transport and communication, food, supporting facilities, analysis of data on tourism, growth of tourism in this territory, views and satisfaction of the tourists are very important to promote the Tourism in a particular place. Each and every aspects of analysation, of discussion, of data is very much useful for the tourists, tour operators, travel agents, tourism organisation, hoteliers, A & N Administration, all govt. officials, researchers, academicians and those who are interested in tourism. After making such a detailed study, how the infant industry tourism could be developed is to be decided and analysed. So an attempt has been made and full attention is concentrated carefully on planning tourism and its overall development in these islands.

Type of Tourism

The first and foremost point to be decided is as to what type of tourism is to be encouraged in these islands. Generally, tourism is classified into Domestic and Foreign. But the classification to be made here is whether rich tourism or cheap tourism. If rich tourism is encouraged, normally, the number of tourists will be less. Income from the tourism industry will considerably increase because the tourists will spend a lot and they would not disturb the normal tradition of these islands. The overall supervision will also be easier. But, whether these islands get always such rich tourism in the long run is the only threat to such rich tourism. Instead, if the cheap tourism is encouraged, more number of tourists will visit these islands. Income from the tourism industry will increase but comparatively at low rate because the tourists will spend less. There are possibilities that the socio cultural tradition of these islands may be disturbed. Then the growth of such cheap tourism must immediately be checked when it begins to damage the original environment or social life of the people of these islands. The carrying capacity of this territory is to be considered while deciding which type of tourism is to be encouraged. It is evident from the tables and discussions in the previous chapters, that the average length of stay is only 7 - 10 days. So the inflow and outflow of tourists are balanced and hence the carrying capacity of these islands is never disturbed. The prediction here is that the cheap tourism will not always be cheap and it is fully hoped that it will not further go to a level of cheaper and the cheapest. So the planning for tourism should be carried out in such a way, that all types of tourists, rich or cheap are to be attracted and they should be induced to spend maximum according to their level of income. The facilities are to be provided in such a way which will suit all types of tourists inclusive of a satisfactory profit. For example, Mr. A, a rich tourist and Mr.B, an economy class tourist visit A & N islands. A would like to spend more and B less. Mr. A & Mr. B are going for shopping and they would like to buy shell made item with the idea(A) to spend more and with the idea (B) to spend less. Suppose, they wish to buy 'Necklace', the island should make available the necklace at the cost of Rs. 1000 per peice which will be preferred by Mr. A with the best quality flaw material and produced by the skilled labour and also another necklace at the cost of Rs.500 which will suit 'B' with good quality raw material. Otherwise a separate shopping complex with the facilities of " Seconds " may be provided so that the economy call tourists may purchase at less cost. Hence, the restrictions on tourism, i.e only rich tourists will be allowed and the cheap tourists will not be allowed to visit these islands, need not be a imposed atleast at the present stage since the Tourism Industry in A & N islands is in its infant stage. All tourists are to be encouraged with the careful planning.

Resource Planning

Planning for tourism development is not an overnight work and that too for sensitive places like A & N islands. All aspects are to be carefully studied and taken into consideration at the time of planning for tourism. Success or failure of the tourism depends fully on how we plan and carefully implement it. While planning, one should not forget that the tourists are the guests who would be discouraged even if there is a small negligence on the part of the planners. It is a very sensitive issue because a dissatisfied tourist would become worst advertiser and a turndown friend who would make the industry sick within no time. At the same time, the Natural and

Man made resources should be protected, conserved and should not be damaged The socio -cultural aspects should not be polluted, damaged and they should also be fully protected and guarded and maintained in such a way the tourists should learn and assimilate the valuable culture of A & N islands.

A & N islands is rich in her resources particularly tourism resources. All are unexploited, unpolluted and under-exploited. Some are studied, enumerated and the rest majority of them are not enumerated and left as they are. 86% of the total area is fully covered with different types of forests by exposing her natural scenic beauty and attracting tourists. Here, people from different regions, religions, different faiths have been living without any difference of opinion. There are good prospects for the tourism but at the same time growth of this tourism industry should not affect the environment, pollute the socio cultural life style of the people of these islands. So effective care must be taken at the time of making plans for the development of tourism in these islands. The tourism resources are to be planned and presented to the tourists in such a way that more and more number of tourists both foreign and domestic tourists are attracted to these islands without affecting the life style of the people of these islands. Hence the experts, academicians and specialists from the different fields are to be called and consulted and the planning for tourism is to be made.

Accommodation

While planning for tourism, what kind of accommodation to be provided to the different types of tourists must be decided. For this purpose, the status of the tourists, income level of the tourists, their possible programmes, pattern of expenditure, foreign or domestic etc., are to be taken into account. Number of hotels which will accommodate the rich tourists are found only in Port Blair city, but the inter-islands do not have such accommodation facility. At the same time, even in Port Blair, the accommodation which may facilitate the stay for middle class or lower class tourists is not enough and totally absent in the inter- islands where the tourists have to fully depend upon the PWD or Forest department guest houses. If any officer is on tour to the other island the possibility of getting accommodation in such guest houses for the tourists will be nil. Tourists are frustrated when they face such problems in the interior places. So a suitable place must be chosen in the important inter islands namely Rangat, Mayabunder, Diglipur, Neil, Havelock, Wandoor, Chidiatoppu etc. and small hotels, rest houses, guest houses, youth hostels, dormitory accommodations preferably with first floor constructed which will suit both domestic tourists and foreign tourists who are at middle level and rich level. As far as the form of ownership is concerned, the A & N Administration may invite the private investors to construct such small accommodation under the overall control of the tourism department in all such administrative matters namely fixing the tariff, provision of facilities, etc.

Another development has been noticed in the growth of tourism industry in these islands. That is the arrival of group tourists and family tourists is more than 10 - 30 persons. Sometimes this number goes beyond 75 also consisting of number of families. They would like to stay in a family type of accommodation. That is big room with kitchen facilities where they would like to cook according to their choice of taste, convenience and homely atmosphere. Once, about 60 persons (employees) came from B H E L of Thiruchirapalli, Tamil Nadu who asked for such accommodation by expressing their willingness that they wanted to stay more days if such accommodation was available. This form of accommodation will be heartily welcomed by both the tourists i.e Domestic and Foreign. While making such accommodation, care must be taken to choose the place which should be near the bank, bus terminus, post office, taxi stand, market etc.

Off-Season Problems

As is already mentioned, the best season for the tourist is from the October to mid of April and the season from mid of April to September is not much favourable for the tourists. In particular, May, June and July are very acute months when the number of tourists is very low. The lodges, hotels and other accommodations are not even 50% occupied during this season. Since there are no private hotels/ accommodations in the inter islands, this problem is not visible to others. Once if the tourism industry is grown, this problem will be obvious, needing a separate treatment. To attract more number of tourists even in this season, the tourism department, hotel owners, lodge owners etc may calculate the concessional tariff and benefits on the basis of principles of marginal costing and announce the same. These concessions may be in the form of :

1. Discount during the off -season periods.
2. Meals on No Profit and No loss basis.
3. Concessions if any tourist stays for more than 5-6 days.
4. Charging tariff for single tourist though they are more than two or three.
5. Family tourists' concession.

6. Sight Seeing/City Tour may be provided freely by the Hotel owners if the tourists stay for more than 5-6 days
7. The accommodation owners may declare that the halls and even big rooms are available for the conference, seminars, discussions, talks etc. at concessional rates so that the institution located nearby and even nearby islands would be using it with some prestige.

So it is suggested that in Port Blair city the accommodation may be provided to the tourists during this off season at a discount of 50% and in the inter islands the accommodations may be provided at a discount of 30%.

Air/Ship Fare

Another difficulty facing the tourists is intolerable air fare and ship fare. Very recently the ship fare as well as air fare have been increased. Even the tourists have expressed such problems. Major part of their total spending goes only for transport and that too while coming from one point to another point, i.e. Chennai - Port Blair, Calcutta-Port Blair, Vishakapatanam - Port Blair. This increasing fare discourages the tourists to come to these islands and hence the tourism industry does not come up. Tourism in mainland flourishes because the transport cost is very low. To travel even 2000 kms. the tourists hardly spend Rs. 200 - 500. So they would like to spend more and more on other shopping items etc. with an intention to stay more days. But in island tourism, a tourist spends Rs. 10,000 - 30000 only on transport just for to and from charges. They are unable to go around the city and spend less because they have to keep another large sum to go back to the mainland. Moreover, the A & N islands is one of the important organs of our mainland of India like North Eastern Hill Regions. There people fly at a very low rate covering almost the same distance. So it is suggested that the air fare and ship fare may be reduced by adopting the technique of marginal costing by merging a marginal margin with the fare. During the off season a 40% discount may be given to the tourists in order to attract more number.

Transport Service

Foreign and Domestic tourists visit these islands by taking leave or with some tight programme schedule. It is quite normal that they may face language problem since they come from different parts of the country/ world. Hence what they do, generally, is that they book / reserve the tickets for their modes of travel in advance and even they book for hotels and other accommodations. But the sudden change of shipping and flight schedule, diversion of ships, cancellation of ships, non arrival of flight from mainland, sudden strikes etc. are the dangerous factors contributing a lot of tension to the tourists. This is because all bookings, reservations of tickets and hotels, accommodation etc. will go waste and moreover they have to stay in mainland till they get their further reservation, if there is a delay on the part of the tourists due to the reasons mentioned above.

It is understood from the discussion with the tourists leaving for Chennai/Calcutta next day that they would like to stay some more days in these islands but due to the uncertainty of shipping schedule, they leave the islands so early. Hence it is suggested to have a regular transport services i.e both Air Service and Ship Service between the Islands and Mainland at the present situation, without any change or hindrance etc.

Introduction of Islands Air Service

At present the A & N Administration is having a separate Shipping Department with a large number of employees. It is having 2 passenger cum cargo ships, 2 cargo ships plying between mainland and islands. As per the available information the Administration grants concession, subsidies and bounties to the Shipping Authorities. It is suggested that the A & N Administration may purchase two Aircrafts(Very New) without any meaningless agreement as happened in the case of the M V Akbar and the same may be operated between Island - Mainland - Island on no profit and no loss basis. Two round trips each to Chennai and Calcutta with a modified fare are suggested. The proposed timings may be as under:

Port Blair — Chennai

Trip	*Departure from Port Blair*	*Arrival at Chennai*
I	04.00 a m	06.00 a m
II	04.00 p m	06.00 p m

Chennai — Port Blair

Trip	*Departure from Chennai*	*Arrival at Port Blair*
I	7.00 am	9.00 am
II	7.00 pm	9.00 pm

Port Blair — Calcutta

Trip	*Departure from Port Blair*	*Arrival at Calcutta*
I	5.00 am	7.00 am
II	5.00 pm	7.00 pm

Calcutta — Port Blair

Trip	*Departure from Calcutta*	*Arrival at Port Blair*
I	8.00 am	10.00 am
II	8.00 pm	10.00 pm

If the Island Air Service is started, it will be a solution for many transport problems, a booster dose to the island tourism, and will be gracious to the tourists and other public from the Administration, and best over of booms. It is suggested that a high power committee consisting of experts, academicians, technicians, excluding politicians may be constituted to invite the offer from the private investors to operate such Island Air Service if Administration so desires.

Provision of Health Service

Still the image of "Kalapani Andaman" in the minds of some public in the mainland dominates and hence it forces them to think about mosquitoes, malaria fever etc. Only very few people understand about this lush green marigold sun paradise Hardly one or two cases are found of malaria and it makes a name as such. So it is suggested that health department of these islands should take all steps to eradicate malaria, Andaman Fever etc. by taking proper steps and as a challenge. Mere going to every house and giving some suggestions will not solve the problem and purpose. The department should find out cause and effect and try to cut at the root cause. The important tourists enter like Port Blair city, Wandoor, Chidiatoppu, Rangat, Mayabunder etc. It is suggested that 24 Hrs. health service should be provided to the tourists. Serving with smile is absolutely necessary in order to develop the Industry.

Instructions to the Private Accommodations

Tourists are very much particular about the place of stay. During the tourist season, really the tourists face problems due to non availability of accommodation in the city and in the inter islands. Though they wish to stay in a costly hotel they are forced to take some cheap accommodation where there is no laundry, laboratory, mosquito net, proper ventilation, protected drinking water facilities and are in bad hygienic conditions. These types of accommodation will make the tourists frustrated and indirectly force them to have a bad opinion about this destination. So it is suggested that the Tourism Department must have a regular checking of all accommodations whether the basic facilities are provided with proper hygienic conditions or not.

Construction of Public Toilets

At present, in A & N islands there is no 'pay and use' toilet. Public toilet facility is totally absent at important beaches like Carbyn`s Cove, Wandoor etc., and parks like Gandhi park and Marina park etc. The road sides and other important place are made dirty due to the want of public toilet especially during the festival time. So it is suggested to construct public toilets with the provision of maintenance at important places of the city, important beaches, grounds and parks.

Construction of Mile Stones and Pillars

A & N Administration may immediately conduct an overall survey in order to fix the mile stones, concrete pillars, sign pillars and plates etc. Each road, street, lane, footpath, village etc. should be rightly and necessarily named. In some islands, places are termed as ' Theen Number' & 'Char Number' etc. Such names may be replaced by some freedom fighters' names. For every 3 Kms. tourist map, made out of concrete plates, of that or nearby locality should be fixed so that the tourists do not face any problem.

Promoting Local Industries

As A & N islands is very famous for the shell made items, wood made items etc., the amount spent by the tourists on shopping directly stimulates the local industries and handicrafts Tourists visit these islands happily and purchase the locally made handicraft items as a symbol of visit to Andamans. They even present these items to their kith and kin, relatives and friends, as a sign/mark of their love and affection with a proud thought that this is made in Andamans. Such purchases by the tourists increase the total efficiency or quality of the local artisans, employment opportunities, the revenue to the islands and economic development as a whole. So it becomes necessary to know the main items or products which are purchased by the tourists both Domestic and Foreign. In A & N islands, there are no silk saree industries, iron industries etc. So the scope of shopping for the tourists is limited to the shell made items, wood made items and forest products. Some sellers charge extraordinary high price from the tourists and such activities of some unscrupulous sellers disturb the shopping behaviour of the tourists and thereby the growth of tourism industry. The tourism department or the A & N Administration may calculate the cost of production of the items which are eagerly purchased by the tourists by adopting the technique of marginal costing technique and ask the sellers to sell only at that price fixed by the Administration. So it is suggested that the A & N Administration may have some control over such local industries by creating a special cell who will look after price control, quality control etc. of the products in which the tourists are interested. Local industries may be guaranteed for the supply of Raw Materials and purchase of final products by the A & N Administration/tourism department.

Protecting the Socio-Cultural Life

The socio cultural life of the people of A & N islands is unpolluted, highly valued and need of this hour at present situation, and just can not be compared with any other region or country. While planning for tourism, care must be taken to protect the socio-cultural life style of these islands. This is because, some religious heads, politicians from different parts of mainland through their talks, create some tension among the people of these islands. The department of tourism should come forward to verify such activities. Talks, speeches by such people on the open ground is not a problem but the way in which they talk and speak which are splitting the people is the problem and that should not be allowed. Hence it is suggested that the clearance from the Tourism Department for such speeches, talks should be made compulsory. Tourism Department should, before granting such permission, take note of their proposed speech and talk and verify them so that it should not affect the growth of tourism industry and should not damage the socio cultural life of the people which is one of the important tourism resources.

New Tourism Routes from Abroad

A & N islands is surrounded by Thailand, Burma, Vietnam, Cambodia, Malaysia, Singapore etc. Air distance between A & N islands and the nearby countries is given below. A tourist who wishes to visit the lush green paradise has to travel a long route or distance by adopting different formalities of international rules. For example, a tourist from Bangkok wishes to visit A & N islands, he has to travel from Bangkok to Calcutta/Chennai and from Calcutta/ Chennai to A & N islands. That is he has to travel nearby about 3500 kms. to reach these islands whereas the distance between Bangkok and Port Blair is just 544 kms. The tourist has to spend for airfare to travel 6000-7000 kms. for to and fro. If there is a direct route to A & N islands, he travels only about 1000 kms. for to and fro and so the expenses come down. In the same manner, a tourist from Japan, has to come to Delhi and from Delhi to Calcutta/Chennai and from Calcutta/ Chennai to A & N islands. If there is a direct route to Andaman from Japan, from Bangkok and so on, the tourists particularly the foreign tourists find it very easy to come to Andaman by saving a lot of amount which can be spent by

Table No 1

Air Distance between A & N Islands and Nearby Countries

	A & N Islands	*Countries*	*Distance (in Kms.)*
1.	Great Nicobar	Atjeh	135
2.	Car Nicobar	Phuket	378
3.	Port Blair	Rangoon	422
4.	Port Blair	Phuket	447
5.	Port Blair	Bangkok	544
6,	Port Blair	Penang	655
7.	Carnicobar	Penang	558
8.	Port Blair	Cox's Bazar	668
9.	Port Blair	Kaula.Lampur	817
10.	Port Blair	Singapore	1011
11.	Carnicobar	Singapore	897

Source: Rajavel 1998.

the tourists on shopping at Port Blair. The tourists from a abroad do not stay for many days and do not spend much in Andamans because the major portion of their expenses goes to transport part. So it is suggested that the Govt. of India may take steps to put the A & N islands on any two international routes as proposed below:

1. Bangkok — Port Blair — Chennai
2. Malaysia — Port Blair — Chennai
3. Chennai — Port Blair — Malaysia
4. Chennai — Port Blair — Bangkok

If such proposed routes are opened, the A & N islands will attract more number of tourists from abroad, Since the distance to be travelled would be reduced by the extent of 5/6th, i.e, 85 % & the traveling expenses also would be reduced to the same extent which will facilitate the tourists to stay for more days by spending more in A & N islands and thereby our country will earn a lot of foreign exchange.

Disposal of Sewage

The Port Blair city, the only thickly populated area in this territory has to be beautified. The first hindrance for the beautification is the stagnant sewage at important places of the city. Gutters do not have free flow of sewage water. Channels of drainage have to be properly designed and constructed accordingly. Nature cleans the whole territory by way of heavy rain. But some senseless persons throw waste, empty bottles, body of the dead animals etc. into the gutters which results in the blocking of sewage. The A & N Administration may announce through AIR and the Daily Telegram Newspaper that the people should not throw such items into the channels of sewage. It may also announce the punishment if they do so Dustbins, litter boxes are to be placed at every 100 meters and regularly the dust bins and litter boxes are to be cleared.

Reservation Facility

As far as the sea transport between these islands and the mainland is concerned, the reservation facility may be made available in the mainland also The S C I and the Directorate of Shipping of A & N islands may recruit some agents at the places far away from Chennai, Calcutta and Vishakapatanam. For example, if a tourist of Kanyakumari wishes to come to these islands he/she has to contact the SCI office, Chennai for availability of tickets, shipping programme and the SCI office or Directorate of Shipping, Port Blair for the reservation If the reservation facility is available in the mainland itself and the agents are nearby, it will facilitate the tourist to take quick decision and action. So it is suggested that the shipping authorities may appoint some of their agents at different places suitably away from the Chennai, Calcutta and Vishakapatanam.

More Islands for Foreign Tourists

At present very limited islands have been opened for foreign tourists. And the foreign tourists are not allowed to stay during night hours in any island. It is suggested that more number of islands may be opened for the foreign tourists.

Lighting Facility for Beaches

Lighting facilities may be provided for the roads which are going to important 1beaches like Carbyns cove, Wandoor, Chidiatoppu etc. and also in the beaches itself. Seating facilities with the decorated shades may be constructed at the centre of the beaches. The centre place which contains the proposed chairs and tables may be fenced and maintained neatly, and be provided with illuminated designed colour lights. Regular checking must be made to check the immoral activities.

Drinking Water

Soft water is another major problem in this territory. Water for drinking is a vital important resource. At present there is only one dam which supplies water for drinking and it is- Dhannikari Dam. But another tank called Thilthaman Tank which was used as a source for drinking water is, at present, used for water sports. But the water sports can be played in any wave-less sea water also. Growing necessity of water, due to the increase in population, for drinking purpose compels the Administration to find out different means for the storage of rain water. So it is suggested that the Thilthaman Tank should also be used for drinking purposes and the water sports may be stopped.

Removal of Fallen Trees

The places like Chidiyatappu, Wandoor etc. are the fine beaches. But they are shrouded by the fallen trees. They have a good quality of soil but with the hidden timber nails of fallen trees hinder the free walk of the tourists on beaches. These beaches are not at all cared by the A & N Administration. These fallen trees have economic value. If they are auctioned, the Administration can get a good amount of income, which can be utilised, for the development of the beaches. So it is suggested that the Administration may take immediate necessary steps to remove the fallen trees from the beaches in order to bring back the beauty of the beautiful beaches.

Cable Cars / Rope Ways

Cable cars/rope ways is an interesting attraction to the tourists. This is the best source of entertainment. At present such cars/rope ways are totally absent in the A & N islands. If this source is provided, it will be like adding honey to the mixed fruit juice. The following places/points are suggested to install the cable cars/rope ways:

1. Haddo to Bambooflat
2. Haddo to Chidiatoppu
3. Mount Harriet to Ross Island
4. Marina Park to Ross Island
5. Wandoor to Redskin/Jollybouy
6. Carbyn's cove to Ross Island

Buses and Bus Terminus

Number of buses must be increased. Since A & N islands is a multi lingual society, the name plates of the destinations should be written in at least four languages namely, Tamil, Hindi, Bengali and English in all the passenger buses irrespective of the ownership. Instructions may be issued to follow this system strictly and regularly. One more bus terminus is to be constructed near school-line. Buses for the places outside the Municipal limit may be operated from this proposed bus terminus, i.e., Long route and very long route buses are to be operated from the proposed bus terminus.

Accommodation at Mainland

Tourist accommodation near the harbour and the airport may be constructed at Chennai, Calcutta and Vishakapatanam which may contain more number of dormitory type beds. This is in order to facilitate the stay of the tourists and visitors of A & N islands. The tourists may be allowed to stay for a period of 10 days depending upon the rush. No tourist should be disturbed with the popular and meaningless words like "VIP is coming, so please vacate". It is suggested that the so called disturbing VIPs may not be allowed to stay in the proposed guest houses and even if they are allowed, they should be treated at par with the tourists so far as they stay in the accommodation.

Possibility of Free Port

These green islands are located on the world maritime route. Particularly the Great Nicobar is very near the route. Though not all, atleast the Great Nicobar Islands may be taken for the consideration of declaration of the opening of Free Port. It is strongly believed/expected/predicted by the author that if the island is declared as Free Port, the A & N Administration will get a lot of revenue in terms of foreign exchange. But this issue is to be properly studied by taking all factors into consideration. So it is suggested to appoint a separate project committee, excluding the political parties, to study the issue.

Others

1. The floating hotels may be constructed in the Port Blair city. For this purpose any scraped shipping vessel may be purchased and used.
2. A&N Administration may invite private sector to run 'pay and use' toilets, bathrooms etc. at important places such as bus terminuses existing as well as proposed, parks, beaches, bazaars, taluk head quarters etc. The tourism department may be entrusted the work of supervision in order to check the immoral activities.
3. Facility of getting the tickets both for ship and flight by post may be provided both in the mainland and in the islands. Necessary arrangements may be made either by the SCI, Directorate of Shipping or Indian Airlines or by tourism department.
4. The Shipping authorities may publish the sailing programme at least, one month in advance in the leading and well circulated daily

newspaper which can facilitate the tourists to make their programme well in advance.

5. Adequate inter islands transport facilities may be provided by the A & N Administration in order to facilitate the tourists to fulfill their programme as per their pre-planned schedule. Regular and adequate inter island transport facility can be a booster dose to the tourism industry which is at its infant stage.
6. A & N Administration should fix the standard price and standard quality for the various food items. This should be strictly followed by all the hotels, guest houses, canteens and hostels etc. Proper feed back should be maintained for the quality control. The standard price should be acceptable by even a lower income bracketed tourists.

To conclude, the A & N islands is a very beautiful tourists destination. It is evident from the survey that the tourists have high opinions about the tourism attractions of A & N islands. The suggestions for the tourism planning in these islands have been offered which are based on the problems facing the industry and the possibility of development of the tourism industry in this lush green paradise.

Conclusion

It is easy to give suggestions, to recommend schemes etc. but the feasibility of their implementation should be taken into consideration particularly from the point of view of finance. By and large, all suggestions, made above, are economically viable and feasible and worth trying. The A&N islands has vast potential resources to be exploited for the development of tourism industry and it is upto the planners and the A & N Administration, Govt. of India, Development authorities to provide more tourism facilities so that the tourism industry will grow to a greater extent which will also contribute to the development of Indian Economy. For that, there should be a wide publicity and advertisement about A & N islands, a provision to show the visitors/tourists a glimpse of the socio cultural life of this Mini India (A & N Islands) and to make them feel that the A & N islands is the place for National Integration in the world. Popular lectures and shows should be arranged in these islands for the tourists who have come to A & N islands and in the mainland for the tourists who are in the mainland to highlight the value and importance of these islands, and the vital role played by the places of interest. What is required is a bold decision by avoiding any to vitalize tourism with the long-term benefits in view in A & N Islands. All these facilities would make the visit of the tourists to these golden sunny Bay Islands, both memorable and happy.

PART III

Education Related Factors (ERF)

1. Higher Education
2. Science and Technology

1. Higher Education

1. Are We Value Oriented?
2. Need for Reformation in Examination System
3. A Study on Academic Freedom in the Quality of Higher Education.
4. Need For Re-Designing The Commerce Education
5. Management of Cooperative Education and Training in A & N Islands
6. Management of Change.
7. How To Conduct Interview?- A Model

2. Science and Technology

1. Concept of Science and Technology in The Economic Development.

23

Are We Value Oriented

Introduction

A fact which cannot be opposed by anyone is that, by birth every individual is an animal and has the nature of the animal. Through the process of education, he is made man. According to Mahatma Gandhi "Education is the converter of the child into man". Education is a unique feature that plays the most dominant role in the life and evolution of humanity. A fully educated man is the real human resource and is considered as an important tangible asset of the country. The socio, cultural, political and economical development of a country depends fully upon such tangible assets. Therefore, we can say that education plays a vital role in shaping and sharpening the personality of a person.

Present Scenario

Both the state government and the central government have been giving more emphasis on the quality of education. Huge amount is allocated every year in the budget for education. However, in practice, the actual expenditure goes beyond the budget allocation. Since such over expenditure is for the development of education, the governments have been granting approval for such excesses. But, the quality of education, as we see, is deteriorating day by day. The cost of education has been increasing without any corresponding increase in quality. The present days' students who have completed their college education are not quality wise equal when compared to people who have completed school education 20 – 30 years ago. Obscurantism, religious fanaticism, violence, fatalism, superstition, untolerable office politics, etc., have become the special features in every organisation and particularly the educational institutions. Now-a-days, the following activities have become almost common features.

Students' unrest, Staff unrest, Dirty politics among the employees particularly among the teachers, unhealthy conflicts among the staff particularly among the teaching staff, leg pulling & spreading grape-wine news, delay in file movements, poor decision-making, improper coordination, confusing communications, partiality and favoritism, strikes & lockouts, absence of work, culture and opposing the superiors, growing arrogant nature and disturbing the society and criticizing the right person and supporting the wrong elements.

The ultimate result of the situation pushes the quality of everything down. The eternal values, honesty, tolerance, truthfulness, coverage, hard-work, loyalty, sincerity, dedication, helping tendency, and other excellent values, of course, cannot be made powerless but they will reach the person and particularly the right person in small quantity due to these present day situation. Dedicated, sincere and hard work officers/employees are not allowed to function properly and are not allowed to live happily. Proper help do not reach the needy persons. in every organisation, one can witness that one group of people will always work sincerely without any recognition and deserving reward. At the same time another group of people will not work at all and they will be sitting idle, buttering the superiors by getting full recognition and even with unimaginable rewards. The third group of people will normally attend the organisations with great confusion of what to do and what not to do? The result will be valueless work, ineffective functions, unproductive expenditure, and criminal wastage of the time and energy.

The Educated

Education, from primary to higher education has been given supreme place because the future of the country fully depends upon the real value of education obtained and absorbed by the educated (students, Parents, scholars, teachers, officers, researchers, administrators, consumers, businesspersons etc.) during the teaching-learning process. Many authors have given many definitions –for the term "educated". But as per my knowledge educated means a person/individual who is involved in the process of learning and has acquired enough quantity and quality of knowledge sufficient to live happily in the society without damaging the happiness of others by facing the challenges before the mankind.

Characteristics of the Educated

I expect the educated to possess the following characteristics:–

Understanding self, common sense and general knowledge, clear-cut communication, respecting others' feelings, understanding the system prevailing, understanding and doing one's work, respecting parents and the other elders, work culture with clear thinking, perfect performance of the allotted duties, punctuality with perfect planning, loyalty towards the job and superiors, God – fearing, innovations and inventions helpful to the society, kind to the society, balanced speech, helping tendency within his ability and budget, open hearted movements, thankfulness and gratitude, taking care of parents particularly at their old age, unselfishness with managing qualities, if teacher, thorough teaching, punctual and discipline without wasting time.

Values

Values are different kinds namely Aesthetic Values, Spiritual Values, Moral Values, Social Values, and Cultural Values and so on. These values are the part and parcel of our life. It is the main ingredient of philosophy. It is the mainspring of the human characters and of the nation and that of its education system. The values are the guides to think and act, program setters, policy makers, Procedure and Rule framers for the accomplishment of the desired goals in the life. In fact values are the principles of the human life, which are the basis for the all around development. A man without any value is considered to be a living corpse. He cannot be regarded as a useful asset but he is lifeless solid state of collection of flesh and bones tied up with nerves. Only the Values make the man full, lively and happy.

Need for Value Education

While comparing the ancient days with the present days, there is no doubt we have gained with certain scientific developments but there is not doubt that the quality of human population has also been depreciating. One should not get angry after going through this article. We should carefully think and analyse the different situations. Are we really happy with what is actually going in and around our country as far as the quality of the human life is concerned? The "Ship" qualities are totally absent. Do we really have friends having friendship? The friends without friendship, the relations without relationship, the partners without partnership, the entrepreneurs without entrepreneurship, the teachers leaders without leadership and heads without headship, the teachers without teacher-ship, the students without studentship, the wardens without warden-ship, managers without manager ship and humans without human ship qualities are the main sources for the today's adverse situation. Little developments coming up in and around our country are only due to the persons with the –ship qualities. For example, in every organisation there are people with sadist qualities, to create tension and problems to the others as well as for themselves. They can never be happy and they cannot give happiness to the others. They cannot understand the good things in a good manner and right things in a right manner. They will always have doubting nature and will try to spread the quality to others also. They might have obtained many degrees but lack qualities in values. The man who has been given the authority to supervise such valueless elements has to devote more time to advice, direct, instruct and to control such valueless elements. However, it will take long time to correct such fictitious assets. The main reason for this is the absence of knowledge about values on the part of the such fictitious assets. So it is considered and seriously thought that there is an absolute need for us to give a proper value based and value oriented Educational System. Even the National Policy on Education highlights the urgent need for value education in view of the growing erosion of essential values and increasing cynicism in society.

What is Value Education?

Education is of different types and kinds. What is going in mass at present is only academic education. People come inside the institution through admission, they buy some books and take the notes from the teacher, get it by heart, retain them till the examination and vomit them through their pens, get marks and they call themselves as educated without understanding the value of education. When they come to the employment market and the society garden they are unable to suit to the society. They do not know how to find a suitable happy life and feel that they have missed something when they were in the educational learning process. That something is value education. So Value Education is an Education which teaches different values, ways and means to live well and happy in the society, to find happiness, to make others happy. This includes – How to live life? How to live happily? How to find happiness? How to make others happy? How to manage all kinds of people? How to manage all kinds of happenings and situations? How to grow and succeed in the right manner?

Now another question that comes up automatically is – Which is more important – Academic education or Value education? We cannot give a correct answer for such question because both are important. Value education is to be carried by the academic education. Both are self-plugging, auto-holding to each other. Without formal education, you will not be able to read or write. Without these skills, you cannot get a good job or manage even the simple things of daily life. Without value education, the academic education has no meaning and at the same time the value education itself can not travel and reach the people. The academic education is a transport that carries the value education to the people. If a highly qualified, well-employed person does not know how to behave properly, does not know how to move with the others, does not know how to understand the prevailing system etc., then his education has been a waste.

Suggestions for Value Education

The governments have been emphasizing more on the quality and the value in the present system of education. It is true that the people take the education buy by ignoring its values and qualities. For example – it is a common feature that a candidate who appears for the interview will be asked many questions during the interview. At that time, he will promise that he will be sincere and dedicated and not indulge in any politics or in any activities which will damage the organisation. In addition, he will promise that he would be punctual and duty conscious etc. These statements are true till he gets job and he will try to keep up the words till he get the appointment order and he will try his level best to remember the promise till he is confirmed in the Post. After that his activities and loyalties towards the job and superiors, behaviour, attendance, quality of the work and dedicated ness would totally change. Therefore, it is suggested that the following measure may be adopted to bring the values in the present system of education.

Value education is not like other academic education that has to be started from the first standard onwards. It can be given at any stage. There must be a separate and special subject on value education and that particular subject is to be made compulsory to all the classes including at graduate and post graduate level of all discipline. Care must be taken to frame the syllabi for such curriculum. Different aspects of values like duty conscious, sincerity and honesty, work, brotherhood, control of anger should be taught from the school level onwards.

Slogans and Writings on the Value of Education and Value Education are to be displayed inside the class room. One should not under estimate the value that will be produced by these slogans. They will not only teach the students but also the teachers, and parents as well.

Conclusion

In conclusion, I wish to say that value education is the real education to be given to our children. To give value education both Teachers and Parents should co-operate with the government. The role of the administrators is very important to impart value education to the young generation. They should posses all the qualities of a true educated. For that purpose, a clear-cut and well defined functional system is to be constructed and to be implemented in the Educational Institution irrespective of the size of the Institution. The head of the institution should not take it lightly. He must be very vigilant in the implementation of the system. The period of the implementation of the system is the period of the incubation of the Value Education to the children. Carelessness of the head of the institution if any will be reflected in the children. The Teachers, Parents and the Administrators are to be very perfect in their duties, responsibilities, sincerity and in discipline. All teachers are to be properly instructed to obey the system. The teachers are to be instructed to go to the classes in time without wasting the allotted time for the class. Teachers are to be properly advised to conduct the tests, quiz, group discussion and all such programmes that will increase the students' talents. Loose talks inside the class with the students are to be totally avoided by the teachers. The teachers/staff who do not obey the system should be brought under severe punishment. The teachers are the models for the students. They should be very careful while talking with the students. The teachers must make the students to know that there is a system and everybody must respect the system. The parents should move with their children freely with the inquiries about the happenings in the institution. When they find free time to talk with their wards, they should discuss the importance of the family, family's position, how to live happily in the society by helping others, without disturbing others, importance of father and mother to the children, what they have to do at their old age, importance of keeping-up the words, patriotism etc. The Administrators have to look into the problems from the social, moral and value point of view. He should not be partial and he should not safeguard the culprits. He should have the courage to face the challenges and the problems created by the worst elements in the organisation. He must organize the meeting with the staff and stress the importance of the value education. So, if the three factors namely teachers, parents and administrators do acquire the characteristics of the true educated, and if a well – designed curriculum is introduced in the present educational system, it is certainly believed and hoped that it is possible to make education a forceful tool for the cultivation of the desirable ethical, spiritual, moral, social, aesthetic and all other eternal values. Such Value Education will create a new generation of individuals or convert the existing unbalanced individuals into individuals with value knowledge, which will help to live life well, to find happiness, to make others happy and to manage all kinds of people and happenings with discipline, honesty, tolerance and truthfulness.

24

Need for Reformation in Examination System

Abstract

The growth and development of education and higher education fully depend upon the extent of the effectiveness in the conduct of Examinations and the system of Examinations adopted by the authorities concerned. The present piece of work concentrates on the existing examination system and its problems in the higher education, prospects, and suitable suggestions to improve, to develop the higher education through the Effective System of Examinations both External and Internal Evaluations. The main ingredients of examinations are the time of examination, completion of the syllabus, intimation about examination and question papers, the method of setting the question papers, quality and experience of the examiners, the conduct of examinations and valuation of answer scripts. Some courses will have house exams; annual exams; external and internal exams; marks for practical and project works and internal assessment marks etc. No proper system is adopted to calculate the internal mark. Some of the teachers who are responsible for giving internal marks do not calculate the internal marks by adopting any base or basis. For the award of internal assessment mark, the tests including practicals, seminars, assignments including practical, quiz programmes, are to be conducted. General behavior of the students including the dressing of the students, number of classes attended by the students i.e the regularity in attending the classes should also be taken into consider for the award of internal assessment marks. But, generally, the importance for the attendance, assignments, seminars, tests, Quiz programs and behavior including the way of dressing etc. is totally omitted in the process of higher education and in the calculation of internal marks. The formula for the calculation of internal marks, responsibilities for the conducts of the above tools have been constructed and recommended in the successful process of higher education.

Education

Education is a unique future that plays the most dominant role in the life and evaluation of mankind. It is important, as eyes to a man, to his life. By birth every individual is an animal and he has the nature of animal. But during the process of growth he is made through education as a man. A man who is fully educated is the real human resource and is considered as an important, a valuable, and tangible asset to the country. The economic development of the country depends fully upon such real assets. Hence, education – Primary, middle, secondary, higher secondary, college including Art, Science, Commerce, Technical, Medicine, Information Technology, Education etc. – plays a vital role in shaping, sharpening and refining the personality of the person. Education particularly higher education has been given a supreme place of special importance because it can provide ideas and worthful human asset to give shape to the future and also sustain to all the other levels of education. Higher education provides a proper solution to each problem of human beings, trade, commerce, industry, social, spiritual, culture, political, agriculture, administration, services, and the quality of overall environment. The growth and development of education and higher education fully depend upon the extent of the effectiveness in the conduct of Examinations and the system of Examinations adopted by the authorities concerned. The present piece of work concentrates on the existing examination system and its problems in the higher education, prospects, and suitable suggestions to improve to develop and the higher education through the Effective System of Examinations both external and internal assessments.

Innovations

Innovation means introduction of something, which is new or different from the existing one. It may be good or bad or neither. As such innovations in education are introduction of merely something, which is new to and different from the existing system of education. It may be the introduction of new system of syllabi, new framework of curriculum, new design of authority- responsibility relationship, modified or new system of management of educational institutions and enhanced learning etc. It may be involved in the improvement in the quality in teaching with refined curricula, reformation in the present system of examination and setting up of question papers etc. Hence, innovations may include the attempts at reforming examinations to improve the standard of teaching, learning and research and the scheme of restructuring of courses, introducing interdisciplinary courses within the general principles of relevance and flexibility. Of all the above, the present system of examination need a thorough reformation due to its drawbacks. So, this paper attempts the innovations in reforming examination to improve the standard of teaching, learning and to improve the quality of education by analysing the present examination system.

Examinations

Examination means a system of device adopted by the authorities by applying on the taughts with a view to promote them to the higher classes. It is a system by, which the students are classified to know the depth of knowledge and memory power retained in a period of 02 and a half or 03 hours. Generally, in examinations all the students are given the same tasks, they are not allowed to consult each other nor they are allowed to refer any books and they are expected to write the answers for the given questions within a given period of time. The answers written by the students are valued and appropriate marks are awarded. By having the norms, the results will be announced with different grades like distinction, first class, second class, third class fail and compartments etc.

Need

Before going to the system of setting the papers, the nature of the examination is to be totally overhauled. In all the universities, the examination system is to be divided into two namely External and Internal Assessments for all the courses irrespective of the classifications such as Commerce, Science, Arts etc. For all the courses, practical curriculum should be included. A thorough and common system is to be developed in the external and internal assessment. Rules and Regulations are to be framed by analysing the problems in the existing systems and they are to be strictly followed and to be implemented. In fact, this is the need of this hour.

Problems in External Assessment

The main ingredients of examinations are the time of examination, completion of the syllabus, intimation about examination and question papers, the method of setting the question papers, quality and experience of the examiners, the conduct of examinations and valuation of answer scripts. But in many occasions the students face the problems, inside the examination hall when they get the question papers due to the arrival of questions from out of syllabus, incomplete questions etc. The students will also face the problems due to the want of some clarifications regarding the usage of calculator, the type of paper to be used, usage of different tables, stencils etc. The teachers who are appointed as Central Superintendent may not be aware of all these clarifications due to the lack of knowledge about the regulations of examination.

The quality of the question papers will depend upon the quality, qualifications and the experience of the examiners and paper setters. The questions from out of syllabus pose a serious problem to the students since it is affecting the students psychological and mental pressure. Sometimes the examiners prepare questions from topic not included in the syllabi meant for of the students for whom he is setting the paper. All the universities in our country do not adopt uniform policy in setting the syllabi, pattern, question paper etc.. Even in each university no uniform policy has been adopted for all the courses. Some courses will have house exams; annual exams; external and internal exams; marks for practical and project works whereas others will not have anything like that. Hence, due to this un-uniform policy in the system of examinations for different courses in each university and in different universities creates problems among the students and hence the results will be the "students' unrest".

Another important point in the present examination system is that who will set the questions? And who will assess the answers and the answer scripts? How will be the scripts assessed? Hence, a proper strategy and policy are to be adopted to make this examination system as meaningful, impartial, purposeful, and free from drawbacks and without making delay. What is the minimum requirement that paper setters should have?

All these unsolved questions are to be found with the suitable solutions in the form suggestions.

Problems in Internal Assessment

Now -a- days, no doubt the teachers are well - paid and hence they are to be expected to work more and they should be called to work more. In the management process, the head of the institution must be bold enough to face the criticisms of the anti-academic critics. He should allot more works within the academic activities. The Teachers of the higher educational institutions are to be compelled to conduct prescribed number of tests, quiz programs, seminars, group discussions and to give assignments to the students. They should be asked to maintain records for the same. Some of the teachers who are responsible for giving internal marks do not calculate the internal marks by adopting any base or basis. They give as they wish without any justification and base. They don't maintain records even. Sometimes they do not conduct the tests, seminars, group discussions etc., and without doing so they put the marks as if they have conducted the tests and seminars etç.. Hence, when inquiry comes, the teachers do face a lot of problems from different nook and corners. Again such unbecoming activities of the teachers affect seriously the quality of higher education.

So, the teachers should give importance to the Attendance, Assignments, Tests, Group Discussions, Quiz Programmes and Dress etc. and hence they are required to conduct the tests. Seminars etc., seriously and dedicatively for the correct internal markings.

Ingredients of the Internal Assessment Attendance

Attendance gives and establishes a close relationship between the teachers and the taughts. The students derive benefits by attending the classes in three ways namely learning the subject, method of teaching and concentration, discipline etc. Both the teachers and the taughts face problems if the students don't attend the classes properly and/or regularly. Repetition of the teaching, fatigue, absenteeism, loss of confidence on the part of the students, unproductive salary etc., are some of the major problems. Carelessness in maintaining the attendance of the students on the part of the carefree teachers will led to the Students' unrest, strike, internal politics etc.. Sometimes it creates legal complications also. So, the attendance is to be given importance. But, in the presence system of education, attendance is given less importance.

Assignments

Assignment is one of the tools to measure the student's performance in subject knowledge, understanding capacity, method of presenting the answer, the level of seriousness in concentration of classes etc.. It can not be thought of simple and light. Giving assignments to the students particularly to the students of higher education would keep them always in touch with the subjects. Multiple assignment system is to be adopted in the class to avoid the duplication work.

Seminar

Seminar is another important device to measure and improve the student's ability, performance, and courage in explaining the subject matter, interpretations in front of the learned persons with in a short period of given time. Seminar helps in bringing out the hidden studentship in him. Seminar enables for healthy arguments and thereby produces a real academician through the innovative ideas. Sometimes the seminar functions like a market for the job seekers (educated young and energetic youths) and job providers. Hence, the seminar is to be made compulsory for the students of higher education. But the students come from different type of family background. The students may not be in a position to talk freely and they may have some shyness to stand before his/her classmates or audience. Under such circumstances, the teachers should adopt some role play technique of teaching.

Quiz Programmes

Quiz programmes are also equally important like assignments and seminars. Quiz programmes help in creative thinking and thereby it increases the studentship qualities in students and thereby increases the general constructive knowledge.

Group Discussions

Group Discussion is one of the methods of developing the students' community. It helps in removing the unnecessary fears and complexes of the students. It establishes equilibrium in the routine life of the students. It brings out many findings when the group of students sits and discusses on a common topic informally formal and formally informal. Group discussion should not be confused with the seminars.

Behavior

The ultimate aim of the education is man making and creation of real man who is created through moral, ethical, cultural, legal, and excellent behaviors of the students. The way of talking inside the class, the way of movements inside the class, the way of dressing while coming to the educational institutions, when attending the classes etc., the quality of concentrating the classes are some of the factors determining the behavior of the students. This is to be taken for the calculating internal marks for the students. Care must be exercised that no partiality is to be shown while awarding mark for the behavior for the students.

Dress

Dress makes a man full. This is not only for the students but also for the Teachers. Teachers are to be very careful while choosing their dress particularly for the class room. The author is certainly not against to any type of particular dress. He is very much particular about the dress of the teacher and taughts inside the class. The way of dressing, the color of the dresses, the activities they do with the special type of dresses with his classmates both inside and outside the class and the institutions can not be just tolerated and accepted by any learned persons. Now a days, almost all the places, the importance to the dress is being depreciated. People think that they can go for any type of dress in any manner. They may give thousand justifications for their committing such mistakes. Such people will come to the higher educational institutions with the day casual dresses and night casual dresses, see through transparent casual dresses, bed casual dresses etc. Teachers should normally not allow such type of dresses inside the classes. For that, they (teachers) should be very careful that they should not come in such type of shabby dresses to the prestigious educational institutions. A teacher is always different from each and every person since he or she occupies the third position in the ithicas & literature (Matha, Pitha, GURU and GOD). No one can simply uttar a word that the teachers are not respected. They were respected, are being respected and will certainly be respected by all sections of the society. While awarding the marks one should take this tool also into consideration.

Suggestions

To avoid the drawbacks and the limitation of the existing examination system and fundamental, constructive and structural changes are necessary and hence the following measures are suggested in the form of innovation.

1. Developing and making the student is an art of the teacher and it is a continuous process. He has to take all such steps to improve him. The teacher must watch the students closely in his performance and other general characteristics. In case of any deviation, it is the duty of the teacher to bring the same deviation into the knowledge of his/ her parents. On this principle only, the parents - teachers meeting are conducted at the school levels. But it is very unfortunate, except few efficient teachers, neither the head of the institution nor the teachers bother about such parent- teachers meeting.

2. A teacher should not think and say the decayed words such as " The higher education students are matured, they knew when to study, I don't want to say anything to them, If he takes very less marks, what can I do?, Why should I do inform their parents?, They are college students, so they can do whatever they want?, In college the students can come with any manner, etc." All these thinks and sayings are lazy-men's brain work. If a student takes less mark, even the teacher need not use hard words to the students. He can very well inform the matter to his/her parents through the Principal/ Head of the Institution.

3. For this purpose, the Principal/Head of the Institution must be a dynamic personality with full knowledge about the Principles of Management. Otherwise, the whole exercise of a dedicated teacher will go waste just only because of the inability, defectives of the Head of the Institution/Principal. So, it is the duty of the State and the Authorities to select a Dynamic Personality with dedicating quality on the development of higher education and the full knowledge about the academic procedures, accounting, laws, income tax, finance, training, delegation and decentralization, positive thinking and approach, and the Principles of Management and Equality. All such qualities are named here as Headship qualities Hence, it is suggested that the authorities may adopt all procedures to find out and elicit the Headship qualities as mentioned above at the time of selecting the Head of the Institution. Otherwise, such defective elements will become a incurable virus to the industrial system.

4. An internal assessment mark of 20% and the remaining 80% for the external assessment are to be fixed for all the courses in every university/institute.

5. For the award of internal assessment mark, the tests including practicals, seminars, assignments including practicals, quiz programmes, are to be conducted. General behavior of the students including the dressing of the students, number of classes attended by the students i.e the regularity in attending the classes should also be taken into consider for the award of internal assessment marks.

6. The marks are to awarded for 100 in each test, assignment, seminar, quiz and behavior. As far as the mark for the attendance is concerned, the percentage of attendance will be the marks for 100. Now there 6 six tools namely, Tests, Assignments, Quiz Programmes, Seminars, Behavior and Attendance. The first four tools are to be conducted more number of times, i.e., 'n' times. Average is to be taken for each tool and hence a total for 600 marks will be obtained. It is to be reduced and calculated for 20 marks. Another confusion may arise, how many number of tests, assignments etc ., is to be conducted and what will be optimum size of the tools to be organised. The following number of tests, assignments etc are suggested as optimum size.

(a) Tests – 03 Per Semester per paper.
(b) Assignments – 03 Per Semester per paper.
(c) Seminar & Group Discussion – 03 Per Semester per paper.
(d) Quiz programs – 03 Per Semester per paper.
(e) Attendance – Percentage of attendance will be the percentage of marks.
(f) Behavior including the way of dressing.

7. To avoid the confusions in the calculation of the internal assessment mark the following formula is constructed and is suggested.

Formula:

Internal Mark for 20 =

{AMnt + AMnq +AMna +AMns +Matt +Mbr}/30

AMnt – Average Marks of 'n' number of tests

AMnq – Average Marks of 'n' number of quizzes

AMna – Average Marks of 'n' number of assignments

AMns – Average Marks of 'n' number of seminars

Matt – Marks for the attendance

Mbr – Marks for the behaviour

8. The responsibility of tests, assignments, seminar, quiz programmes attendance and the behavior including the way of dressing are to be fixed with the concerned subject teacher. He has to plan and organize the above programmes in consultation with the HOD (Head of the Dept.).

9. He has to make a written plan of and a copy of which has to be submitted to the HOD (Head of the Dept.) and he has to organize the seminars and the group discussion only in the presence of the Head of the Dept. The concerned subject teacher should maintain a separate register for the conduct of tests, seminars, assignments etc., subject to the inspection of the Head of the Department or the Head of the of Institution. He has to record the date of tests, assignments, portions covered in tests and assignments, marks awarded for the same. It is also suggested that the concerned teacher should take the signature from the students in the register itself. In case of any difference of opinion from the students' side, this record will be the authenticated documents as a proof. The lecturer/teacher

should clearly write the way, the base of calculation of internal assessment marks.

10. Implementation of the system of internal assessment mark may invite some objections from some of the teachers due to the new system of working though not over burden. So, it is highly suggested that the system of internal assessment mark is to be implemented by moral suasion and by adopting the principles of management of change by defrosting the problem creating teachers. The necessary authority with the responsibility must be delicated to the heads of the department or the senior most person in the department concerned.

11. The Principal or the Head of the Educational Institutions should not under any circumstances, interfere in the authority and the responsibility granted to the Heads of the Department.. However the Heads of the Institutions may consult without giving any advice but by offering suggestions to the HODs, if he wants to make any change. At the same time, the Heads of the Departments must be made very clear about the consequences which he is going to face if any malpractice is found in the authority and responsibilities granted to the them by the Heads of the Educational Institutions.

12. The Lecturers/Teachers of less than 10 years teaching experience are, generally, are not allowed to value the papers. The teachers/ lecturers of less than 15years are generally not allowed to set the question papers.

13. Only those lecturers who have completed 10 years of teaching experiences may be given the valuation work and those who have completed 15 years of teaching experiences may be given the work of setting the question paper. The concerned authorities should not have any compromise in this matter.

14. A List of teachers who have completed more than 10 years experiences and 15 years experiences is to be prepared by the head of the institution. For counting the experience, the date of initial appointment is to be taken. The list is to be under the custody of the head of the institution. It is his duty to send the name of the teachers for valuation and for the paper setting in such a way that everybody is getting chance. A same teacher should not be allowed to go for valuation continuously for two years. Atleast on or two years gap must be there.

15. Before the valuation starts, the chairman has to discuss very clearly about the way, methods and techniques of valuing the answer scripts.

Valuation of the papers should not be like a horse race. The answer papers are to be studied & read thoroughly and then the examiners have to assess the marks to be given to each question.

16. Time for valuing each paper is very important. On an average the examiner must take atleast 10 – 15 minutes per paper. Hence, every examiner is to be given 25 Answer Scripts to evaluate in a day of 06 hours valuation. To bring the efficiency, correct judgment and to increase the quality of education, the examiners should not be allowed to work more than 06 Hrs. daily in the Valuation work. The following timings are suggested.

0900 Hrs	—	1000 Hrs	05 Papers
1000 Hrs	—	1100 Hrs	05 Papers
1100 Hrs	—	1110 Hrs	Tea
1110 Hrs	—	1200 Hrs	05 Papers
1200 Hrs	—	1400 Hrs	Lunch
1400 Hrs	—	1500 Hrs	05 Papers
1500 Hrs	—	1600 Hrs	05 Papers
1600 Hrs	—	1630 Hrs	Statement Preparation

17. Number of examiners may be increased with reframing the valuation fees structure. At present the valuation charge for the UG Courses Rs. 6.50 per paper and for PG courses it is Rs. 9.00 per paper. It can be reduced to Rs. 5 and Rs. 7 respectively. Some universities pay very huge amount for the valuation of the assignment papers. If the restructure the valuation fees schedule, they can charge less fees from the students. Uniform pattern is to be adopted.

Conclusion

Once the impediments in the path of the System of Examinations in the Higher Education are removed, and an effective strategy is formulated in the light of the suggestions given, and if the same is implemented carefully through the dedicated and qualified academicians without the yes masters, butter-men, and with out the interference of the political and other unwanted factors and with full meaningful principles, the quality of higher education will certainly improve and will contribute a lot to the over all economic development of India.

25

A Study on Academic Freedom in the Quality of Higher Education

Abstract

There are excellent, dedicated and expert teachers. The concept of academic freedom is very important but it is misunderstood by the teachers(not by all). Academic Freedom means that the teachers should be given freedom to teach the students in the class according to his own style of teaching, as per his own methodology of teaching. Some teachers (not all) commit mistake in the name of Academic Freedom by misunderstanding the term and they created anti-academic atmosphere inside the class. The wrong perception of the teachers about the Academic Freedom is ranked and tabulated. As a result of the misunderstood academic freedom, the head of the institution will find very difficult to control the staff both teaching and non teaching, and the students as well. There are dedicated teachers, hard workers with excellent behaviour and discipline. The teachers should accept whatever the subjects allotted by the head of the department. The teachers should evaluate the workings of the students carefully. Teachers activities are being copied by the students. How to overcome the problems due to the misperception of the term Academic Freedom is given. For the high quality of education, it is necessary that everybody must understand the real meaning of the term academic freedom and the teachers are to be provided with minimum requirements. This is important to convert a normal student into a real human asset.

Introduction

Every head of the institution has been facing problem in the controlling function of managing the institution. This is partly due to the inadequate infrastructural facilities and partly due to the absence of work culture in the institution. If the head takes the institution to the objectives, nobody recognizes him and one cannot find anybody to say atleast a word of praise. But at the same time if there is any problem, there are thousands of people to find fault upon him and talk lakhs of ill on him. A head of the institution can successfully manage the institution if his superior understands the style of management of the head and extends the possible support in the administrative system. But generally every one has known what is going. Majority of the educational institutions fails only because of failure of the head of the institution due to his inefficient management. Majority of the heads fail only because of the absence of the administrative support by his superiors, absence of the work culture on the part of the staff both teaching and non teaching and the defective decisions taken by top management. The staff particularly the teaching staff expects freedom, which is already there but is misunderstood by them. In the name of academic freedom they commit number of mistakes and they become the examples of future generations. By taking the academic freedom as the key point a study has been conducted to strengthen the quality of Education and to stress the work culture on the part of the teaching staff.

Education

Education is a unique feature that plays the most dominant role in the life and evaluation of mankind. It is important, as eyes to man, to his life. A fully educated man is considered to be an important real human resource and hence, he is a tangible asset to the country. In fact, the economic growth and development of a country fully depends upon such real assets. Education both at lower level and higher level has been given a supreme place of special importance because it can provide ideas to shape the future of an individual, society and the country as a whole. Higher Education provides suitable measures to each problem of human being, and hence it is the basis for the culture, trade, commerce, industry, agriculture, political, management and administration and quality of overall environment. So such education is to be given to the growing, innocent and undisturbed minded children.

Present Scenario

The children acquire the name, student when they are admitted in the educational institutions. They are fresh minded, innocent in nature, and excellent in behaviour. Their brains are like unrecorded cassettes and their IQ will be always more. It is the duty of the teachers and other academic staff to make such innocent but active fresh minded children as a meaningful excellent human asset of the country. This is possible only if the teachers train them systematically with discipline. There are excellent, dedicated and expert teachers. But the number is very less. At the same time there are teachers without taking the teaching work as serious. They create hell of situation. They are the bases for the indiscipline. It is unfortunate that the quality of teaching, teachers' behaviour, the method of teaching, extent of clarifications, discipline on the part of the teachers, the quality of the dress of the teachers, the style of dressing by the teachers, the style of language used by the teachers inside the class are being depreciated and deteriorated day by day. Such deterioration strongly affects the quality of education and it becomes the base for the future generation.

Absence of discipline on the part of the teachers, not going to the classes in time, not clarifying the doubts inside the classes, loose talks with the students, criticizing colleagues in front of the students and inside the classes, not conducting test, seminars, group discussion, quiz programmes, non maintenance of attendance and discipline are becoming the normal features of the higher education in the present days. Unhealthy arguments with the seniors and higher authorities by the teachers and other academic staff started increasing more particularly in government institutions due to the assurance of the job securities. Another pathetic condition is that the thinking of the teachers, as " they are very busy" if they go to the classes always late by 20 to 30 minutes of the 45 minutes class duration. They don't maintain proper records for the attendance, marks for the tests, records for the internal marks. They don't obey for the system. Talking always about others inside the institution to earn the sympathy of others is their normal nature and unchangeable characters. They spread a lot of grape-wine news. As a shield, such people use the term Academic Freedom to confuse others by confusing themselves. They misunderstood with the term academic freedom. The concept of academic freedom is very important. But it is very unfortunate that the term academic freedom is used to create unhealthy academic atmosphere in the institutions.

Misunderstood Academic Freedom

As is already mentioned that the term Academic Freedom is misunderstood by the teachers(not by all). They try to give a different meaning for the term "Academic Freedom". The teachers expect that they should not be asked to go to classes in time. They expect that whatever they do in the institution, the head must approve. They expect that all their dues are to be paid in time and sometimes even before the due. They expect that they must be allowed to criticize anybody and everybody in any manner. They ridicule and pass bad comments on the dedicated teachers. Moreover they expect the students should not ask clarifications for their doubts particularly inside the classes. Such teachers expect in the name of academic freedom, the head of the institution must give all sorts of work except the work for which he is appointed. May be the money motive , the reason. Such teachers successfully will do all the non-academic works. All these things can not be claimed as even a freedom. If the head of the institution or the head of the department calls for the explanation on why he has not engaged the classes, they blast like anything by combining some other staff who are also in the same category. So it has become necessary to give a actual meaning of the term Academic Freedom.

Academic Freedom Meaning

Academic Freedom means that the teachers should be given freedom to teach the students in the class according to his own style of teaching, as per his own methodology of teaching. He can explain by taking any number of examples, which are not opposed to public policy and not support to any political party. He is permitted to take any examples but such examples should not create or induce any immoral or illegal in the minds of the students. The teachers should not be ordered to teach only by adopting a particular style or method. Teacher should be allowed to express their views, ideas and solutions to solve the problems of macro level. The academic freedom also means the teachers should not be controlled directly or indirectly to carry out their research work and in publishing their write- ups in journals of national and international level. The teachers are to be allowed to participate freely in the seminar, debates on national and international problems. But it does not mean, the teachers can go to such seminars, workshops by canceling or foregoing the classes. That is the teachers should not to go to such seminar and debate by forgoing the teaching work. He must think that his primary work is to teach. Under any circumstances, a teacher can not and should not forgo the classes. He has to go the classes in time and sincerely teach in the classes.

A teacher can go and attend all such seminars, workshops which are organised after the class hours. That too he can not go in the name of Academic Freedom without telling or informing the Principal or the head of the department. He has to necessarily inform and obtain the permission from the head of the department or from the Principal. The Principal / HOD also must verify and ensure that the students will not suffer if he/she is permitted to go for the seminar or workshop. It is also necessary to mention that the teachers are freely entitled to get all facilities and encouragement his class room teaching, research and his attending seminars and debates. Many Experts and Dedicated Teachers have already defined what an Academic Freedom is. So, this is called Academic Freedom but at present some anti- activities are confused with the term and are claimed as Academic Freedom.

Data Analysation

By seeing the Quality of the Education particularly the higher education, a pilot study was conducted to know the real reasons among the 15 students First the reasons and causes are identified. Then it is decided to make a questionnaire to find out the views of the mass. 150 Students of different disciplines have been selected for the study. A semi structured questionnaire was prepared and served on them to know the causes. Out of 150, only 139 questionnaires are received back. Even among 139 questionnaires, only 113 questionnaires were fully attended. Rests were more than 60% incomplete. Hence, the 113 questionnaires were taken for the analysation purpose. Some facts were elicited from the from the pilot study. All such facts and information collected from the Pilot study are very dangerous in nature and slow killing poison in practice. Some teachers (not all) commit mistake in the name of Academic Freedom by misunderstanding the term. These facts were included as questions and asked in the questionnaire.

Going to the institution regularly late by twenty to thirty minutes, Going to the classes regularly late by fifteen to twenty minutes in a period of fifty to sixty minutes, Leaving the class regularly ten to fifteen minutes before the completion of the period, Leaving the institution by forgoing the classes to attend his personal works. Conducting No Class Test, No Seminars and No Assignments, Writing personal letters inside the class, Passing bad comments about the other teachers and self boosting, Only dictating notes without explaining about the subject, Going on writing on the Board without explaining the subject matters, Covering one chapter in three months and ten chapters in one month, Taking tea and snacks during class hours, Asking the students to go for the remittance of electricity bills, telephone bills, cell bills etc. during the working hours, Sitting with the head of the institution and head of the department by forgoing the class without any care and seriousness on the classes and Impartial award of marks in the internal assessment etc., are some of the serious issues.

All these problems and issues cannot just be taken lightly. In actual sense, these are the basic bases of the students' unrest and staff unrest. It is understood that all the above transactions are claimed as the rights and academic freedom by some of the teaching staff. The views of the respondents are given in the following tables.

Table No 1

Views of the Respondents on the Activities of the Teachers.

S.No.	Views of the Respondents & Activities of the Teachers	No. of Respondents Told Yes	No.	No Comment	Total
1.	Teachers come to Classes always late.	87 (77.0)	17 (15.0)	09 (8.0)	113 (100)
2.	Teachers leave the classes Always early	76 (67.3)	28 (24.7)	09 (8.0)	113 (100)
3.	Personal Work inside the classes	64 (56.6)	42 (37.2)	07 (6.2)	113 (100)
4.	No communication about the Classes.	89 (78.8)	22 (19.5)	02 (1.7)	113 (100)
5.	Talking irrelevants inside the Classes.	69 (61.1)	42 (37.2)	02 (1.7)	113 (100)
6.	Making comments about the Other Teachers inside the classes	47 (41.6)	39 (34.5)	27 (23.9)	113 (100)
7.	Teachers do not explain the subjects in the classes always.	62 (54.9)	23 (20.4)	28 (24.7)	113 (100)
8.	Teachers do give only notes in the classes always.	69 (61.1)	44 (38.9)	-- --	113 (100)
9.	Talking too much Personal Experiences in the classes	66 (58.4)	29 (25.7)	18 (15.9)	113 (100)
10.	Covering the Portions at great speed	91 (80.5)	22 (19.5)	-- --	113 (100)

11.	Going on writing on the board & irrelevants inside the classes.	76	17	20	113
		(67.3)	(15.0)	(17.7)	(100)
12.	Comparing teachings of other teachers inside the classes	66	29	18	113
		(58.4)	(25.7)	(15.9)	(100)

Table No 2
Ranking of Wrong Perception about Academic Freedom

Sl. No	*Wrong Perception About Academic Freedom*	*Ranking*
1.	Covering the Portions at great speed	I.
2.	No communication in & about the Classes.	II.
3.	Coming to Classes always late.	III.
4.	Always writing on the board	IV.
5.	Leaving the classes always early	V.
6.	Talking irrelevants inside the Classes.	VI.
7.	Giving only notes in the classes always.	VII.
8.	Talking too much Personal Experiences in the classes	VIII.
9.	Comparing teachings of other teachers inside the classes	IX.
10.	Personal Works inside the classes	X.
11.	The subjects are not explained always in the classes	XI.
12.	Making comments about the teachers inside the classes	XII.

Table No.01 clearly shows that different types of activities are totally confused with the academic freedom. The teachers expect that they should not be asked for anything including why he has not gone to class. When they reply for these questions, the students showed their feelings by explaining their real problems they face. Some teachers have created such an anti-academic atmosphere inside the class that they (teachers) can whatever they feel to do. Some students do not want to say anything due to the fear of leaking the information. They reluctant to give their opinions inspite of the promise about the data collection i.e "the data collected will be used only for research work and will be kept totally secrete." It is understood at the time of data collection that the students have more knowledge on the common behaviour than that of some teachers who have wrong perception about the academic freedom.

Table No. 02 is related to the ranking of the wrong perception of the teachers about the Academic Freedom. Generally the teachers do not have the work schedule as far as the planning for teaching is concerned. The teachers do not evenly take the syllabus of the subject for the teaching. During the initial periods of the reopening of the institution, the teachers do take lightly of going to the classes. They show that they are very busy in all things except teaching for which they are appointed. Then at the last moment, they will come to the classes and say the headings of the syllabus of the subject and coolly declare that the portions are over. 91 representing 80.5% of the total respondents expressed that the teachers cover the portions at a greater speed. They cover one chapter in two months and ten chapters in one month.

Another serious problem is that the teachers do not communicate both about the classes and subjects inside the classes. Whether the teachers will come to the class or not, whether the classes will be engaged or not, Tests will be conducted or not and nothing will be communicated to the students. The students will have to sit till the last hour without any work and finally they have to leave the classrooms. 89 representing 78.8% of the total respondents have expressed this problem. While expressing the problems, the student respondents told that the teachers do not come to the classes in time and also they leave the classes well in advance 87 respondents with 77.0% and 76 respondents with 67.3% of the total sample have expressed these problems. 09 respondents with 8.0% have not told anything and they were silent by without giving of their comment. Another misunderstood academic freedom is that their personal works inside the class without teaching, comparing his teaching with other teachers' teaching, giving only notes inside the class without explaining the subjects, and talking irrelevants like passing comments about other teachers, talking personal experiences inside the class etc. Sixty-Four respondents representing 56.6%; 69 respondents representing 61.1%; 66 respondents representing 58.4% of the total sample have expressed that the teachers have misunderstood the above as their freedom.

Problems

As a result of the misunderstood academic freedom, the head of the institution will find very difficult to control the staff both teaching and non teaching. Due to the job security in the government jobs, the staff talk too much rules and regulations. Moreover the misunderstood academic freedom adds fuel to the burning fire. Since the teachers (not all) go to the classes always late and leave the classes early, go on giving the notes without teaching, talking irrelevant inside the classes, passing comments about other teachers, and other unbecoming activities of the teachers inside classes and the institution in the name of the academic freedom will seed the indiscipline among the students community. For thinking it may be very light but in the long run this will create a big problem to the Nation as a whole. Every such teacher will find difficult to control the students and they can not teach well even after correcting themselves. The misunderstood academic freedom on the part of the teachers will spoil the society in different angles and it will become a chronic problem to the educational world and no one can find solution for such problem in future, if the corrective steps are not taken now.

Suggestions

Tc remove such misunderstanding about the academic freedom, the teachers are to be very clear about the their duties and responsibilities. What they have to do and what they are not supposed to do ? One should not simply say that he knew every thing. Thinking like this is the first step of misunderstanding the Academic Freedom. In the light of the above discussion, the following measures are suggested to remove the misunderstanding about the Academic Freedom.

1. All Teachers do not misunderstand the term Academic Freedom. There are dedicated teachers, hard workers with excellent behaviour and discipline. But there are anti academic elements also present with the problem creating behaviours in the institutions. The head of the institution must identify them first. If he (head of the institution) fails, then everything will fail.
2. The head of the institution must conduct the meeting of the staff and clearly explain the duties, responsibilities, accountabilities, powers and rights of the teachers. He should not forget to say the consequences if the teachers do any ultra vires activities. The head of the institution must clearly make them to understand that their primary work is to teach.
3. Every teacher must think sincerely that he is appointed to teach the students, Teaching is his prime duty. Under any circumstances, the teacher should not think that teaching is burden to him. If so, he has to understand himself that he must resign the post and to leave the institution. The teachers should not be allowed to do any work by forgoing the class or classes. This is the work of the head of the institution who must carefully watch while allocating the work.
4. The head of the institution must not be partial and he should be bold to face the challenges and the reactions of the bad elements. He should not help anybody against the Rule.
5. The teachers must be provided with all facilities which will increase their efficiency to contribute more to the students in the institutions. Each teacher must be provided with the following:

(a) A small room or a partition in a big room
(b) A Table and Chair with additional two chairs.
(c) A three feet Steel Almirah
(d) A computer with Printer
(e) Library Card with the right to draw minimum of ten books.
(f) Right to conduct the seminar in the afternoon i.e after the class hours.
(g) Right to consult and to be consulted and to express his views.
(h) Right to get all his dues monetary and non-monetary in time.
(i) Right to publish his research findings whatever it is and, but his popular thoughts if they are not against the public policy.
(j) Right to participate any Seminar/Workshops/Special lecture etc. after the class hours(0900 to 1530 Hrs.) without the permission of the head of the department or the institution.

6. Some of the important Duties & Responsibilities of the teachers are:

I. The Teachers must be present in the institution in time i.e at the starting hours. He should not be under any circumstances late to the institution. In the same way he must be present in the class in the class hours. He should not go to the classes late even by 05 minutes. The teachers must wear good looking dresses and casual dresses should not be permitted insider the classes.

II. Teaching sincerely the undergraduate and postgraduate Classes as per the syllabi given by the Head of the Department. The teachers should accept whatever the subjects allotted by the head of the department. There should not be any arguments and the head of the institution must not and should not interfere in the work allotment process by the head of the department. The mere fact is that the Master Degree Holders should be able to teach any subject in the curriculum. Even if they have not studied in their course, they are supposed to prepare and teach. Teachers must coordinate and cooperate with the departmental activities as is required by the Head of the Department.

III. Supervise the research activities of graduate and undergraduate students and assist in the supervision of students/ research projects at a postgraduate level. Teachers should not have any loose talks inside the class rooms. They should not under any circumstances talk or pass comments about the other teachers. The head of the department or the institution must view it very seriously. If he fails, it will lead to the students and staff unrest.

IV. The teachers must undertake an active, appropriate and viable personal research programme or participate in team-based research. Teachers must explain the points inside the class and they should dictate any notes. Also they should not rewrite on the board. They have to teach in such a way that they can understand fully and they can write themselves. Such capacities are to be developed by the teachers. For this dedication is important.

V. Publish papers or other scholarly works in academic journals and review papers and the like. Participate in community service activities that further advance the profession or field and which are consistent with the University's/College Charter and Strategic Plan.

VI. Assist the Department to develop an environment, which gives effect to the discipline in the department and the college as well. The teachers must maintain a full record of tests, assignments, seminars, group discussions and other curricular activities conducted by him in the class along with the marks awarded. The teacher should not be partial in awarding the marks. The teachers should evaluate the workings of the students carefully.

VII. Serve on Institution committees as per the requirements of the Head of the Department and Institution. Ensure the observance of Institution system & policy and codes of practice in all teaching, research, community service and administrative practices. Contribute to the development of a Department working environment of teamwork and cooperation.

VIII. The teachers should not do any personal jobs/ works inside the classrooms. Teachers activities are being copied by the students. If they do so the future of the students will be spoiled. So the teachers must be very careful in the process of their teaching.

IX. Any other duties as required by the Head of Department.

Conclusion

So, Education is a unique feature that plays the most dominant role in the life and evaluation of mankind. A fully educated man is considered to be an important real human resource and hence, he is a tangible asset to the country. In fact, the economic growth and development of a country fully depends upon such real assets. Teachers are the base and basis for all officers including administrative officers, doctors, engineers, teachers, pilots, economists, scientists, writers, journalists, authors, workers, principals etc.,. They are responsible for the Nation Building Project in the society. If they are good every thing will be good and the vice versa is also true. There are excellent, dedicative, and hardworking teachers but at the same time there are few academic pathars (rice-less paddy) create hell of problems by misunderstanding the term academic freedom. The facts elicited through the survey may be very simple to think but such facts are like diabetics which will leads to many complicated problems in future. If proper care is not taken in time, such diabetic facts will paralysis the whole body of the institution and the education system of the Nation. So the head of the educational institutions must be very cautious and he is the person who has to identify such pathars and give proper treatment. He must make a strategy in the light of the suggestions given above. Once, if it is made and carefully implemented with the help of the dedicated teachers, the student community will be able to stand in the society as real human asset and resource, which is the basis for the economic development of any country.

26

Need for Re-Designing the Commerce Education

Introduction

Education is a unique future that plays the most dominant role in the life and evaluation of mankind. It is important, as eyes to a man, to his life. A man who is fully educated is the real human resource and is considered as an important, a valuable, and tangible asset to the country. The economic development of the country depends fully upon such real assets. Hence, education – Primary, middle, secondary, higher secondary, college plays a vital role in shaping, sharpening and refining the personality of the person. In the Human Life Cycle the "Education" has been given a supreme place of special importance because it provide ideas and human resource to give shape to the future and also sustain to all the other levels of education. Higher education provides a proper solution to each problem of human beings, trade, commerce, industry, social, spiritual, culture, political, agriculture, administration, services, and the quality of overall environment. The growth and development of education and higher education fully depend upon the extent of role of parents, family, administration and the state. Education, by the curriculum wise, is divided in the Science Education, Technical Education, Arts Education and Commerce Education. The present piece of work concentrates on the existing Commerce Education - its problems and prospects, need for the redesigning and suitable suggestions to develop and to improve the Commerce Education.

Why Commerce?

The students interested in commerce have a wealth of opportunities open to them. Even a region or country with aboriginal set-up, both aboriginal and non-aboriginal set-up or transmission from the aboriginal set-up to non-aboriginal set-up, the commerce-based education prepares students to work in both an Aboriginal and non-Aboriginal setting. "The country Saskatchewan has a strong history of economic development among its First Nations communities. Students with a commerce education are in high demand to lead the organizations to a prosperous future." But now the situation is lightly different particularly in our country that the candidates with the commerce education are considered at par with the non commerce candidates to do all works that are to be done only by the candidates with commerce education. That's why the cost of products has been increasing due to the extra training; unproductive wages for long period to understand the commerce practices.

What is Commerce Education?

Many people still, they confuse the term "Commerce" with the term "business". At macro level, the Commerce and Business are one and the same. But at micro level commerce is a part of Business. That is, the Commerce is one of the ingredients of the Business. Business includes Industry and Commerce. But actually both the Business and Commerce are the branches of Economics. Economics decide what to produce? How to produce? Who will produce and when to produce? Industry helps in converting the raw materials into finished goods with the factors of production and the Commerce helps the such functions by transferring the finished products, by financing such activities, by storing and saving from the loses, by giving the information about the goods & services and by activating the buying and selling the produces, products and services. Hence Commerce includes Finance (Banking), Transport, Insurance, Storage, and Advertisement & Publicity. All activities and transactions such as the how to manage, how to prepare accounts, how to bring the relations with the other factors, how to plan, how to organise, how to direct, how to select the personnel, how to control, how to coordinate, how to communicate, how to report and how to budget & estimate etc., related to the Banking, Transport, Insurance, Storage, Advertisements & Publicity are all called commerce activities and the education about such actions and transactions is called Commerce Education.

Ingredients

The Commerce Education is a very vast in its scope. This is the base for all actions in the human life. All activities totally depend upon the commerce education. As far as the function is concerned, the commerce education includes Planning, Organising, Directing, Staffing, Coordinating, Controlling, Communicating, Reporting and Budgeting & Estimating. As far as the areas are concerned, it includes Banking, Financing, Insurance, Transport, Storage, Advertisement and Publicity. As far as the activities are concerned, the commerce education includes Bargaining, Purchasing, Storing, Supplying for Production, Transporting, Selling, Accounting, Analysing, Interpreting, and Estimating. Many people including the officers at higher level think that commerce education means only B.Com and M.Com. But in fact that is not true. Accounts, Management, Costing, Income Tax, Computer Education, Secretaryship, Works, Finance, Marketing, Cooperation, Entrepreneurship, Administration, Banking, Auditing, etc., are all the branches of the Commerce Education. As such, M.Com, MCA, MBA, ICWAI, ICAI, IFCAI, ICS, BBA, BCS, BCA, Diploma in Business Management, Business Administration Financial Management, Personnel Management, and management education of any kind are one way or other related to commerce education.

Present Scenario of Commerce Education

Presently the Commerce Education is given from the Higher Secondary Level onwards. That is from the Plus One onwards. Two years commerce Education is followed by the Graduation Level in the name of B.Com Degree Examination and the same goes upto the Research Degree of Master of Philosophy(M. Phil)and of Doctor of Philosophy (D. Phil or Ph. D). As far as the quality of the Commerce Education at present is concerned, it is not that much satisfactory. The main reason for this is the methods of teaching the commerce education to the young and energetic wave-less brains. The methods need improvement. To examine the quality of teaching the commerce education at plus two level and at degree level both at Graduation and Post Graduation Level a personal visit has been made to few Schools and Colleges. The students were asked questions and the teachers were also interviewed informally. Though the fact, which was the result of the personal observation from these institutions, may not be taken as the universal fact and one should not come to a conclusion that everywhere the same practice is going. There are excellent institutions and teachers who dedicate themselves to the commerce education. But the facts recorded by the personal observation are true. The followings are the result of the observations.

At Higher Secondary Level

The teachers write on the board all the questions and answers both in theory part as well as the accounts practicals part. The teachers don't explain the terms, definitions, and the concepts. They ask the students to write the written answer in a register and submit the same as if the students of their own write it. Some teachers compel the students to come to them for special coaching in the name of Tuition and thereby they earn more money. Even in tuition, they dictate the questions and answer and ask the student to mug-up (by heart) the same. Yet, Some teachers lack the capacity of teaching and they find difficult to teach the accountancy subject and other syllabi. The students also practice by heart without knowing the actuals of the subjects.

At Graduation and Post Graduation Level

The teachers/lecturers do not go to the classes in time. Some teachers lack the capacity of teaching and they find difficult to teach the accountancy subject and other syllabi. The teachers don't explain the terms, definitions, and the concepts. The lecturers use stage talk generally and come back. Some teachers teach accountancy as theory subject without writing on the Board and theory as accountancy subject completely writing on the board. They write even a definition on the block board at degree level and at the PG level. These techniques are nothing but passing time inside the class. Some teachers take the notes, prepared by them 15/20 years ago when they were the students, to the classrooms, dictate and comeback. Number of developments might have taken place. How much difference must have been in the data during the year 20 years back and data of today's developments that are not made known to the students.

Yet some teachers and lecturers will never go to the classes by taking Class IV jobs in hand or by taking some excuses. They will concentrate more on all such jobs except for which they are appointed. The subject which is to be taught in 90 Periods will be taught by him in 09 periods by showing he is very busy in developing this universe. They will pretend and act as sincere teachers in front of the Head of the Department and Institution. The actual and ultimate sufferers are the poor students. Such teachers always have a sayings as a shield "They are PG Students and they will study themselves" The Tests, Assignments, Seminars, Group Discussions, Quiz Programmes etc., are the part of the academic works which will not be conducted by the teachers and some teachers (not all) will produce the list of marks and records as if they have seriously conducted the Tests, Assignments, Seminars, Group Discussions, Quiz Programmes etc.

Defective Curriculum

Commerce Education is, actually, a professional course. Due to the deterioration in the quality of the commerce education, and defective curriculum construction and design, it is now being placed at par with the other conventional pass degree courses. The management education, accounts education, secretaryship education, entrepreneurial education, computer education etc., have been started as separate faculties by diluting the commerce education. The teachers and institutions alone cannot be blamed for such lacunas arise in the quality of the commerce education. The curriculum was designed as per the needs of those days when commerce education was introduced.. But still the same style, structure, inclusions etc have been followed, of course, with the light changes. At present, it does not include the syllabi that are very important and required by the society.

Number of talks are going to remodel the curriculum but it is in vain. The course design is not consistent. For example, syllabi for the Higher Secondary Course, Degree Level and Post Graduate Level are not constructed in a consistently advancing way. Lot of repetitions is there. In Degree Level and Post Graduate Level the portions are very less and every year the volume of portions are reduced. The system of examination is also defective. The question paper pattern also does not contain the instrument to examine the analytical capacity of the students. There is no practical work in the commerce education at present. The curriculum does not include or compel the field project work. During the interview and discussion, it is submitted that the students do copy the reports of the previous year and that's why the field project works are not introduced. It is not the mistake of the students and it is very well the laziness of the teacher and head of the department and institution. The heads must bring the necessary rules and regulations to have the proper feed-back.

All universities do not follow the uniform pattern of the syllabus. The standard is not fixed, level of understanding the subject is not estimated, required knowledge whether expert knowledge, general knowledge, practical knowledge, executive knowledge etc., is not determined. Even if they are fixed, constructed and determined, it is not followed strictly. Even in accounts the very important practical chapters are not included. Students pass out without knowing about the particular chapters. The Students find it difficult to do a problem in a simple calculation of average due date which is very well in practice now. The main reason is that the average due date is not included in any of the commerce curriculum except one or two universities in their distance education programme. All such drawbacks of the present commerce curriculum make the commerce education defective.

Need for Redesigning

Commerce Education has its number of major roles to play in the process of economic development of our country. Commerce Education is a Common Education, it is the Education for Business . Commerce is the basis for all ultimate activities. Commerce is absolutely necessary for Business, Small Business Opportunity, Business Bureau, Business Plan, Business To Business, Business and Economy, Small Business Grant, Small Business Administration, Business Service, Internet Business, Home Business Opportunity, Business Yellow Page, Business and Finance, Business Software, Starting A Small Business, Business Directory, Sample Business Plan, Business School, Investor Business Daily, Business Franchise, Business License, On Line Business, Business Idea, International Business, Home Base Business, Small Business Association, Home Based Business Opportunity, Small Business Idea, Commerce Business Daily, Business News, Business Consulting, Computer Business, Business Search, Business Ethics, Business Intelligence, Business Proposal, Business Management, Business Journal, New Business, Business Web Hosting, Business Suit, Small Business Financing, Internet Home Business, Web Business, Writing A Business Plan, Business Advertising, Business Development, Business Phone System, Business Start Up, Business Magazine, Internet Business Opportunity, Business Planning. It includes almost all the activities of the human life. So, No life is without Development, No Development is without Business, No Business is without Commerce and No Commerce is without Commerce Education. Hence, the Commerce Education is a primary need of every country. A meaningful commerce education will take the country from the underdeveloped stage to the developing stage and from there to the economically developed stage. Hence, Right from the higher secondary course, the commerce education is to be carefully designed and curriculum is to be rightly constructed.

Redesigning

As is already pointed out that the Higher Secondary Level (+1 & +2), the commerce education is being taught at present. In + 1, there are two papers called Business Studies and Accountancy. In + 2 also there are two papers in the same name. Syllabi for these papers are not consistently designed and constructed. Many portions are repeated. The pass out students who are seeking admission into B.Com or BBA etc., have to study once again the same subject, same portions and such practice makes the students lazy, carelessness not only in their course but also in their lives. For example, Sole Trader Final Accounts, Partnership Accounts, and Company Accounts are in +2 and the same is repeated in B.Com and BBA etc., Though the standard differ from the +2 to Degree, the students do practice and the teachers also do teach the same manner and finally the examiners also set the question papers in the same manner. Some students face problems in doing simple mathematics at the degree level and even at the post graduate level in commerce education. But they do not study even a simple mathematics and statistics at +2 level commerce education. They come out with the same level and disturb the future students community. These type of practices dilute the importance of the commerce education by making wasting the years as far as the education is concerned. Hence the following redesigning is suggested for the commerce education.

1. The name of the Commerce Education is to be changed into Business Education. The abbreviation B.Com Degree is to be replaced by the abbreviation BBS which means the Bachelor of Business Studies and the M.Com by the MBS which means the Master of Business Studies.
2. The Plus One and Plus Two are the bases for the Commerce Education and at present two commerce papers are taught in the name of Business Studies and Accountancy are to be continued but the syllabi are to be changed. In plus one in the Business Studies paper the following syllabus is recommended. Principles of Business, Principles of Management, Principles of Business Environment, Principles of Banking, Principles of Transport, Principles of Insurance, Principles of Storage, Principles of the Advertisements and Publicity.

Factors of production, Office Organisation, Theories of Management, Management Thoughts, Institutions related to business.

3. As far as the Accountancy in Plus one is concerned the following syllabus is recommended. Definition and Accounting Cycle, Principles of Accountancy, Functions of Accounting, Accounting Standards, Concept of Accounting,, Views about Accounting, Groups interested in Accounting and Why? Features of Accounting, Terms of Accounting, Preliminaries in Accounting, Books in Accounting like Sales Day Book, Cash Books, Bills Receivable Book, Payable Books etc., Models of the Books, Limitations of Accounting, Uses and Importance of Accounting- Difference between the Accounting and Accountancy, Book-keeping and Accounting, Double Entry Book Keeping System - Classification of Accounts, Journals, Journal Rules, Ledger, Debit, Credit, Account, Balancing, Assets and Liabilities, Capital and Investments, Income, Expenditure, Receipt, payments, How to write journal, How to write date etc., Nature of Income, Need for measuring the Income, what is Cost, Revenue etc. Trading and Non-Trading organisations. Trial balance, Profit and Loss Account, Balance Sheet. How to open a Bank Account and How to maintain the Bank Account? Preparation of Cash Book, Pass Books, Bank Reconciliation Statement, Rectification of Errors, Bills of Exchange, accommodations bills, Receipts and Payments Accounts.

4. As far as the plus two is concerned, the Business Studies Paper must include the following Chapters. Functions of Management – Planning – Organising-Staffing- Communicating- Controlling – Coordinating – Reporting and Budgeting -in detail, Financial Management and Marketing Management in detail. The Accountancy paper must contain the following chapters. Sole Trader Final Accounts, Accounts related to Average Due Date and Account Current, Depreciation Accounting in Detail- Accounting for Sale or Return Basis- Self balancing and Sectional balancing – Single Entry Book Keeping System.

5. Level of Teaching is to be very thorough. Students are not to be asked to mug up (by heart). The principles are to be ciearly explained with many examples. Strict discipline is to be maintained.

6. A simple Project work is to be introduced with the practical problems of a data collection with the Sole traders and other non trading

organisations and they may be asked to draw the final accounts of the concerns.

7. As far as the Degree Level is concerned, the commerce education i.e the proposed Business Education is to be divided into 10 specialised groups given below. Each group consists of three Subjects as Optional I, II & III. Each Subject is to be taught fully in V & VI Semester as Paper I and II. The students have to take any one group.
   (I) Advanced Accounts and Income Tax
   (II) Finance and Audit,
   (III) Banking and Insurance,
   (IV) Marketing and Salesmanship,
   (V) Computer and Internet,
   (VI) Secretaryship
   (VII) Costing
   (VIII) International Trade and Transactions,
   (IX) Organisation and Management, Office Organisation,
   (X) Rural Development and Village Administration,

8. As far the Degree is concerned each year must have 10 Papers and if it is semester pattern, each semester will have 05 Papers.

First Semester

(a) National Language (ONE)
(b) International Language (ONE)
(c) Basic Business Mathematics,
(d) Business Economics
(e) Business Law Paper

Second Semester

(f) Business Correspondences
(g) Financial Accounting Paper I
(h) Costing Accounting
(i) Business Environment
(j) Management Information System

Third Semester

(k) Marketing
(l) Principles of Business Management

(m) Financial Accounting Paper II
(n) Business Statistics
(o) Business Related Institutions

Fourth Semester

(p) Banking Theory and Practice
(q) Import and Export Procedure
(r) Inflation Accounting
(s) Human Resource Development
(t) Research Methodology

Fifth Semester

(u) Indian Economy (Trade, Commerce and Industry)
(v) Field Study Tour –Report (Compulsory)
(w) Optional I Paper I
(x) Optional II Paper I
(y) Optional III Paper I

Sixth Semester

(z) Society and Business (Current Affairs)
(a) Project and Viva Voce (Compulsory)
(b) Optional I Paper II
(c) Optional II Paper II
(d) Optional III Paper II

9. As far as the Post Graduate Business Education, it must have 10 papers each year and if it is semester pattern, each semester must have 05 papers as follows. Each Semester will have one paper common for all Specialisation and the remaining four papers are from the Specialisation. The first year vacation is to be utilised for a On-the-Job training for a period of 31 days in any organisation by having a tie-up programme and the students will submit a Training Report. The final semester will have one paper Research Project with Viva Voce. Hence the syllabus frame work will be as follows:

First Semester

(a) Entrepreneurship
(b) Optional Paper I
(c) Optional Paper II

(d) Optional Paper III
(e) Optional Paper IV

Second Semester

(a) Organisation behaviour
(b) Optional Paper V
(c) Optional Paper VI
(d) Optional Paper VII
(e) Optional Paper VIII

Third Semester

(a) Research Methodology (with Quantitative Techniques)
(b) Training Report (Vacation Period Training)
(c) Optional Paper IX
(d) Optional Paper X
(e) Optional Paper XI

Fourth Semester

(a) Business and Related Laws (with Current Affairs)
(b) Project and Viva Voce
(c) Optional Paper XII
(d) Optional Paper XIII
(e) Optional Paper XIV

For Accounts Specialisation	For Finance Specialisation
Principles and Practice of Accounting	Principles and Practice of Finance
Advanced Non Corporate Accounting I	Merchant Banking
Advanced Corporate Accounting I	Financial Services
Advanced Non Corporate Accounting II	Forex markets
Advanced Corporate Accounting II	Global Financial Markets
Accounting Theory	Income Tax Law and Practice
Bank Accounting	Indirect Taxes
Income Tax Law and Practice -I	Financial Auditing
Income Tax Law and Practice – II	Financial Institutions
Inflation Accounting	Management of funds
Human Resource Accounting	Investment Analysis
Cost Accounting- I	Portfolio Management

Financial Auditing	Financial Management- I
Management Accounting	Financial management - II
Responsibility Accounting	Financial Accounting

For Marketing Specialisation	**For Banking Specialisation**
Principles and Practice of Marketing	Principles and Practice of Banking
Marketing Research	Bank Management
Product Planning and Product Policy	Banking Accounts
Marketing People	Banking Personnel Management
Consumer Behaviour	Management of Funds
Marketing Mix	Investment Analysis
Strategic Marketing	Portfolio Management
Marketing of Service	Consumer Behaviour
Commodity and Exchange Market	Banking Regulation Act
Promotional Management	Bankers Training
Office Management	Financial Management
Personnel Management	Financial Accounting
Finance Management	Human Resource Development
Advertisement and Salesmanship	Mercantile Law

table continued .....

For Costing Specialisation	**For Computer Specialisation**
Principles and Practice of Costing.	Principles and Practice of Computers
Management Information System	Computers and Business
Financial Accounting	Computer Programming - I
Advanced Cost Accounting – I	Computer Programming – II
Advanced Cost Accounting – II	Tally Package
Management Accounting – I	Internet and Intra-net
Cost Management	Computer Language – I
Product and Service Management	Computer Language – II
Cost Accounting and Budgetary Control	Software Management

Working Capital Accounting	Hardware Management
Inflation Accounting	Management Information System
Responsibility Accounting	Financial Accounting
Service Accounting	Human Resource Management
Income Tax Accounting	Principles of Costing

For Management Specialisation	**For Rural Development**
Principles and Practice of Management	**Specialisation**
Financial Accounting	Principles and Practice of Rural Development
Office Management	Public Relation Management
Financial management	Public Finance
Human Resource Management	Managerial Economics
Financial Management	Indian Economy
Stress Management	Agricultural Prospects
Product Management	Small Scale Industries
Quality Management	Village and Kadhi Industries
Public Relation Management	Village Administration
Marketing Management	Panchyati Raj
Management of Funds	Financial Accounting
Foreign Exchange Management	Meetings and Resolutions
Investment and Portfolio Management	Govt. Orders and Policies
	Village Developments

10. The syllabi for each subject are to be carefully constructed. For example, in Accounts and Income Tax Specialisation, Advanced Financial Accounts Optional I, Advanced Cost and Management Accounts Optional II and Income Tax Law and Practice Optional III. Advanced Financial Accounts must have the complete syllabi of the Partnership Accounts, Company Accounts, Government Accounts, Farming Accounts, Electricity Accounts, Educational Accounts, PWD Accounts and like. Advanced Cost and Management Accounts must have the complete syllabi of the Cost Accounts and Management Accounts including the Capital

Budgeting. Income Tax Law Practice must have the complete syllabi of the Income Tax law and practice.

11. The level of knowledge in the Degree Stage (BBS) is Executive Level and the level of knowledge in the Master Degree Stage (MBS) is the Expert Level including the Executive Level. In Master Degree, only the Optional Subjects will be studied with advanced problems at expert level.

12. Each subject is to be taught atleast for a period of 90 Hours in a semester. This calculation is made on a simple Glass Door Method. Total number of days in a year is 365. This is reduced by the 52 Sundays, 09 Second Saturdays, 60 Days Vacations, 15 Days Inter Break, 19 Declared Holidays, 10 days for Annual Day, Sports Day, Seminar Day, Other Functions and hence a net and solid number working days come to 200 constructive days. That means every institution must have 200 working days in a year and 100 Working Days per semester with out spoiling the Effective Teaching – Learning Hours (ETLH). By giving a provision of 10 hours (i.e 10days per teacher and hence for a subject) for the casual leave and other unforeseen leave etc., it is calculated that each subject is to be taught atleast for period of 90 Hours in a semester. The responsibility of monitoring the ETLH is vested with the Head of the Institution. In case, in any subject the ETLH is reduced, the Head of the Institution will be held responsible and he is liable to all the monetary losses both for the management and for the candidates.

13. Each Subject in the Commerce Education and the Proposed Business Education must have the Assignment Work, Seminars, Tests, Group Discussion, Paper Corrections, Strict Attendance, etc. and the concerned teachers are fully responsible to the Head of the Department. The teachers are required to maintain a Students Ledger by recording all the marks awarded to the Students with the countersign of the Head of the Department.

14. No one can skip the classes under any circumstances. If he is given any extra work by the head of the institution or by the head of the department, he has to perform the extra work only after the class hours. Sometimes the teachers will be assigned with some works like election enumeration , liaison duty, survey works and the like by the

government. The teacher cannot take a plea that he cannot go to the class because of the government has assigned some duties. The number of classes a particular teacher skipped is to be calculated and the concerned amount of the salary for the period he/she has not performed the duty of teaching is to be arrived and the same will be deducted from the salary.

15. The Commerce Education and the Proposed Business Education at Degree level ie B.Com & BBS are to be Paralleled and to be considered at par with the Inter Pass Degree/Diploma of the Indian Institute of Management and the ICA, ICWA, ICS, IIFT, etc. as the case may be. The Master Degree of the Commerce Education and the Proposed Business Education ie M.Com & MBS are to be Paralleled and to be considered at par with the Final Pass Degree/Diploma of the Indian Institute of Management and the ICA, ICWA, ICS, IIFT, etc. as the case may be. Hence, the Master Degree Holders of the Business Education/Commerce Education are to be allowed to practice as a Chartered Accountants if their Specialisation is Accounts & Income Tax, practice as Cost Accountant if their Specialisation is Costing, practice as a Company Secretary if their Specialisation is Secretaryship and like.

16. The related rules are to be made that the posts of Accountants, Cashiers, Clerks, Supervisors, Assistant Managers, Deputy Managers, Managers, General Managers, Directors, Auditors, Head Of The Sections, Head Of The Institutions, Head Of The Organisations, Committee Chairmen, Leaders, Secretaries, Directors, People Responsible For Making Policy, Programmes, And Rules; are to be filled up only with the candidates who have the qualifications of BBS & MBS (B.Com & M.Com). The rules are to be implemented strictly irrespective of the government sector, private sector or semi-government sector

Conclusion

The future of any country fully depends upon that country's economic development which in tern depends upon the trade, commerce and industry on one side; the technological development, the entrepreneurship qualities on the other. These factors will contribute to the developments only and if there is proper management with planning, organising, directing, controlling, communicating, coordinating, reporting and budgeting, and with the thorough understanding about the principles of factors, management, financing, transport, storage, insurance and advertisement and publicity etc. An education which has been catering to the above needs is the commerce education i.e the proposed business education. The parents, family, administration and the state have their own shares of responsibilities in the development of such education. Generally the family is responsible for a combined decision making in youth among the small group of persons. Next to the family, the teachers play a very important first hand role in shaping and molding the students' carrier in higher education. But at the same time the role of administration is equally important in planning, organising, directing, staffing, communicating, and controlling and in coordinating. The state is the supreme power in providing higher education to its population by providing and establishing the educational institutions at all level. The state is the policy maker and decision making authority regarding the establishment of higher educational institutions and the educational standard because it is the finance provider. Even in the educational management also, the commerce/business education plays its effective role.

Once the impediments in the path of the present curriculum of the commerce education are removed, and an effective strategy is formulated, and the commerce education is redefined and the new subjects introduced with the practical aspects in the light of the above suggestions given, and if the same is implemented carefully through the dedicated and qualified academicians without the yes masters, butter-men, and with out the interference of the political and other unwanted factors and with full meaningful principles, the quality of Commerce/Business Education will certainly improve and will contribute a lot to the over all economic development of the country.

27

MANAGEMENT OF COOPERATIVE EDUCATION AND TRAINING IN & AN ISLANDS

And another article on Management of Change

(Please See in Part II Business Related Factors (BRF) under Trade, Commerce and Industry)

28

How To Conduct Interview?- A Model

Introduction

Interviews cannot be done in a monotype for all the jobs. The style and process of the Interview is to be changed for one job to the other. The method of Interview adopted to select a clerk or even an officer cannot be adopted for the selection of a lecturer or a teacher. This is again true in case of a teacher and the principal; Cashier and head clerk and so on. What are employers looking for in employees? What traits are considered valuable? Are very important variables to be taken into consideration? For that purpose, the employers have to carefully select the Interviewers (IVRs) rather than the candidates for the Post. The quality of the interviewers will definitely reflect in the selected candidates. So the selection of interviewers is the major task of the employers. If the employers really want excellent human assets to work with the principles of esprit de corps, then they have to select meaningful team of the interviewers. Otherwise, the whole exercise will go waste along with the wastage of hard earned money, wastage of time not only for the employers but also for the candidates in terms of candidate hours. It is the duty of the interviewers to select a right candidate for the job in the interview for which they are appointed. But now what is going at present is entirely opposite to a normal expectation of both the employer and the candidates. So an attempt has been made to give a model of conducting fair interview so that the right candidate will be selected for the right job.

Present Scenario

The candidates will be preparing for the interview in hours together, days together, and even months together by spending a huge amount in the books, journals and magazines etc.. But now a days, we all are experiencing that the selection of the candidates are being made by a group of some people in the name of Interview Board, Selection Committee, Selection Board, Screening Committee etc., consisting of may be in two or three or even in upto seven in number in the name of interviewers. But how are they selected for the board ?, whether they follow any norms for the selection of such members for the selection committee etc ?. are the real questions with no answers. All such so called selection committee members with a lot of highly inflated thinking will come to the closed room and they will perform their work. They will ask the peon, normally stands outside, to bring the candidates one by one and start firing the candidate with non stop bullet questions without giving time to the candidates to reply. Moreover, there will be competition between themselves (so called board and selection committee members) that who had asked more number of questions and who had made the candidate tired.

Normally whoever it is, there will be an interview fear and fever with slight tension to every candidate. Due to this non stop firing questions, the candidate will be pushed to go to Coma Stage in the Interview Board and can not even open his mouth and finally will come out. The selection committee members at the cost of the employers will enjoy this meaningless drama. Another pathetic condition is that some times, the questions will be asked by a member who does not know and can not give answer for the same. Some times, another suicidal problem is that a member who has not studied and does not know anything about even abcd…of accountancy will ask questions in advanced cost accounting. Yet another problem is that the serious, real and dedicated candidates cannot tolerate the unrelated questions from the IVRs just for fun. Questions about life and love history of actress, actor, cricket players, play writers, drama writers, name of the novel books are the unwanted questions and unrelated questions for any type of interview. No one can justify that these questions are important to the interview. The candidates will be irritated when they are asked such questions in the interview and they will totally loose their confidence about themselves and on the higher education etc. All these things are going just because of the unqualified IVRs. Such IVRs will neatly submit the report as "Non Found Suitable", or "by selecting his own candidates" and "as per the instruction of the administrators, politicians and his superiors etc".

The term Interview is made out of the words - Inter + View like the words "international", "intermarriage", "interface", "interdependent" etc…. That means all views of a person/candidate. In interview what are all should be checked and examined is yet to be understood by the interviewers. All views of the candidate are to be carefully examined. But the Interview itself is not an end or deciding mechanism. This is because, anything can be manipulated in the interview. If the IVR wants to confuse the candidates, he can very well do it and at the same time if the IVR wants to help the candidates, that can also be done in the interview. So what is required is a sensible, real literate, balanced educated, un-influentiable, dedicated, real educated, impartial, high knowledge and aged gentleman (those who do not drink, smoke kill the office time by chit chat,..) is to be given the authority to select the right candidates. Of all the IVR must know the purpose for which the candidate is going to be selected and he is going to select the candidate.

Problems

It is the normal practice that the selected candidate will say as " the interview was excellent". The unsuccessful candidate will say, as "it seems that they have already notified the candidate". No one can know what has actually happened inside the four walls. If the right candidates are being selected, the productivity, potentiality, quality, speed-ness etc., will improve. But now a day, what is actually going everywhere, every one of us knew it. The delay, bribe, slow movements of the file, non-cooperation, office politics among the staff, staff unrest, insubordination, Griping at others, criticizing, blaming are the common features of almost every institution particularly the government owned. The main intangible reason is that failure of the Interviewers in discharging their duties and responsibilities in a real way. Their failure to conduct the interview in the process of selection is the responsible factor.

Absence to systematic process is the main reason for such problems. One of the most common feelings towards interviewing is fear. It is a shared emotion affecting both the interviewer and the person being interviewed. The interviewers often fails to understand that their main function, duty and the responsibility is to select a right candidate. What mistake they commit is that as soon as the candidate enters the room, they start firing the candidates with the non-stop questions. The candidate will, there itself, loose his confidence about the interview and his selection, and all his subjects and preparations. The funny things are that the interviewers will ask the questions for which they themselves cannot give the answer and they do not know the answer. Normally the interviewers have some peculiar type of disease that as soon as they come to know that they have been appointed as the interview officer, they used to fly by keeping their heads on the air. They prepare themselves as if they go for a battlefield with a view to face the enemies. Some interviewers prepare themselves as if they are going to cut the goat in a festival. Actually the candidates are to be allowed to show their publications and they should be asked to give a presentation. But what is going at present is deadly against this. They omit this important part. Even when the candidate himself come forward to present about his publications etc., due to their weakness, less knowledge about the research publications, pre-influential - bliss, supreme delight, confusion, perplexity and influential-sickness - the interviewers do not want to see and do not want to react upon the presentation. Generally in the name of interview they do not be very serious about for which they have been selected and appointed. They will kill the candidate by asking some irrelevant questions like who was the intimate friend of Mr. X, a famous cricket player, when he was the student of III standard? Do you know the place in Kashmir where one of the Tamilians got married with a foreign girl during 1919. What was the name of the Picture produced in 1900 in which there was a song with the first sentence as Thil Mayin Keeya hai?. This is what, actually, going in majority of the interviews. The interviewers are more careful to confuse and avoid the candidates rather than selecting the right candidates for the job.

Suggestions: How to Conduct: A Model

Before the recruitment and selection, the employers have to be very clear about the type of the job and requisite qualifications and qualities of the candidates to be selected for the job. This is because the employers do invest their hard earned money in the business. So right persons are to be selected for the job.

1. The employers must know the objectives of the interview.
2. Selection of the Interviewers,
3. What is actually expected from the candidates?
4. Steps to be followed during the interview by the interviewers.

Objectives of Interview

The following are the objectives of the interviews. Both the employers and interviewers must know about this and they are expected to be very clear about the objectives. They will have to bear in mind in each and every activity in the process of the Interview failing which the whole exercise will go waste.

1. To give the essential facts about the job and the institution to the candidates.

2. To judge the language fluency in conversation.
3. To see the research publications and the published books
4. To see the candidates' self-assessment towards the fitness of the job.
5. To find out the reason for leaving the previous job and join the new job
6. To get a real feel of the candidate
7. To judge the problem-solving and, difficult situation handling techniques etc., and
8. To judge the physical and mental fitness of the candidate to the Post.

Selection of Interviewers

The Quotation of Brain Tracy is to be verified from the candidates. Because now a days this is very important since majority of the institutions, organisations and units fail only because of such officers who have self centered thinkings of vested interest and more substantial interest. His Saying is "Successful people are always looking for opportunities to help others. Unsuccessful people are always asking, 'What's in it for me?'" Such unsuccessful people are to be rightly identified and they are to be removed list of interviewers. With the great techniques, the employers have to select the interviewers. In fact, this is the first and foremost work of the employers when they are selecting the Interviewers.

What is to be Expected?

Every employer is interested to have an excellent candidate to be selected for the post of for which he is called for. Though the science is considerably advanced, the present days,, are of rush and hurry with impoliteness . The esprit de corps of the workers has been coming down. Comparatively, it is more in the government sector. Hence, it is also one of the reasons for the privatisation. So the employers appoint the interviewers to select the right candidates. It is the prime duty of such interviewers to look and judge the intrinsic qualities of the candidates. So actually what is expected by the employer from the candidates appearing for the Interview is Good attitude, knowledge about the product and the company/ organisation and ability to work hard. It is the duty of the IVRs to check properly in the interview whether the candidates have these qualities or not.

A good attitude

This is the first expectation of the employers that the selected candidates should have the good attitude. Because these days are fast going with rush and hurry. The people with politeness, skills and ability to communicate well with others are very less. Moreover, it is very difficult to find out such people. The employers expect that the selected candidates are to be fit for the team work and the employers are looking for those with the ability to work well with others. It means respecting the thoughts and opinions of coworkers. But Griping at others, criticizing, blaming, or being known as "difficult" is not okay in today's workplace. Smiling, communicating well, and knowing how to be gracious and flexible are the good attitude of the good employees. Employers consider a positive outlook and enthusiasm as important for the job as well as taking responsibility for one's actions and personal integrity. Employers are looking for employees that they can trust, and whom they believe will do a good job. Self-esteem and confidence are considered part of a positive outlook. Employees with a good attitude will contribute towards reaching the company's goals, and adapt well to the culture of the workplace. So the interviewers must seriously check whether the candidates have the good attitude as required for the job.

The ability to work hard

Ability to Work Hard is the need of this hour. Mere knowing the work will not be sufficient in the present day situations of complexities etc. Every employee must think that the organisation is basis for their life and hence they have to work hard to keep the life giving asset always in a developing and growing level. This probably comes as no surprise, but the hard working and productive employee is highly valued by employers. This means being willing to do occasional overtime when required, or doing your best work and not taking frequent breaks or "goofing off" when on the job. So the Interviewers must carefully select the candidates with the ability to work hard.

Product knowledge

Employers expect that the employees must have full knowledge about the Product of the organisation. Here the product means service also. They think that if the employees' full knowledge about the product only can bring the organisation up. Employers value the employee who takes an interest in their company, and understands thoroughly the product or expertise that is the basis of company profits. They also consider enthusiasm and a high opinion of the company and the position, positive qualities. The job seeker can demonstrate this enthusiasm and interest in the company by doing "homework" before a job interview, researching the company, its products, its client base, and possibly having ideas on marketing or increasing production. So the interviewers have to examine the extent the knowledge about the product.

Steps

The following steps are recommended to all the interviewers to get the best candidate for the post for which the whole process is being carried out.

1. The Interviewers have to invite the candidate while he is coming inside the room/cabin where the interview is conducted. He must be invited with smiling faces. The interviewers should not show that they have more power to ask any questions as they think. There is nothing wrong if the interviewers ask the candidate to take a glass of water. The interviewers must create an environment inside the room so that the candidate must feel that he is very comfortably accommodative. It is the responsibility of the Interviewers to bring such situation and atmosphere, then only they can be called as successful interviewers.

2. After having created a accommodative atmosphere, the chairman of the board of interviewers must start asking once again the candidate's name, father's name, father's occupation, his marital status, native place, place of educations, universities the candidate has crossed till date in his education, the present job, his extent of satisfaction in the present job, salary particulars of the present job. As far as these questions are concerned nothing is related to his personal in which he may hide or feel uncomfortable to give answer. Suppose, the candidate came from very far away place or the place of interview is a new one to the candidate, under such circumstances, the interviewers must ask the candidate about his journey – which train he came? How was the journey? Where is he put up at present? Whether he stays with out any problem etc.

3. A fact that is often overlooked in interviewing is that you, as the person conducting the interview, should lead the way. While asking these questions, if the other interviewers would like to join, no problem, they can also very well join. The main purpose of this step is to break the ice. The interviewers must bear in mind that the fear in the minds of the candidates has to go. This step is very important step, because, here only maximum interviewers commit inexcusable mistake. While asking such questions, the interviewers should not

laugh or should not do any visually physical movements that will induce the feelings of the candidate to think that the interviewers are ridiculing. If the interviewers behave in such a way that the candidate feels that he is being ridiculed, then the purpose of the interview will fail and the whole exercise, money, time etc., will go waste.

4. Since, this paper is related to the higher education, and the interview will definitely be related to the post of academic or administrative. That is for the post of Lecturers, Teachers, Readers, Associate Professors, Assistant professors, Professors, Principals, Head Masters, Vice- Principals, Directors or Deputy Directors, Assistant Directors, Administrative Officer, Coordinators, Educational officers, Educational Commissioners, Assistant Coordinators, Secretary/ Manager of the Educational Institutions and the like. The interviewers must again and again keep it in their mind that they are going to select academic and administrative staff.

5. Another important aspect is that the interviewers must converse with the candidate only on the matters in which they themselves and the candidates are very thorough. They must feel that they are impartial, justice, balanced, non-supportive, optimistic in selecting the right candidates, free and frank in the interview board to express his views about the right candidates and to invite the expressions of the interviewee, The interviewers should not allow others to influence them, they should not have any idea to harass the candidate. Because in the interview board anything can be done since it is conducted in a closed door. So what the author wants to stress here is that the right candidate is to be selected for the right job.

6. The next step is that the interview officers must ask the candidate for their academic excellence. Where he got his Secondary Education, Senior Secondary Education, Degree, Post Graduation, Research and Diploma etc.? What are the names of the universities, and the institutes etc., another important question is that the extent to which the candidate has the knowledge in computers.

7. The next very important aspect is that the interviewers have to ask the candidates to present a brief about his fitness, according to the candidates, to the post for which he is attending the interview. Majority of the interview officers/ interviewers do not ask this. The candidate must be allowed rather called to show all his Research Publications, Books Publications, Seminar Speeches, All India Radio

Speeches, and Additional Duties Administered by the candidate and the different Special Positions Occupied by the Candidate. This is the major part of the interview. The interviewers have to judge here only the Capacity, Quality, Qualifications, Potentiality, Productivity, Morality, Mortality, Qualities of Leadership, Capacity to Control, Effectiveness to Plan, Ability to Organise, Direct, Communicate, Coordinate and to Report, Possessiveness to Budget the Activities and Able- ness to move with the others. If they do so then, the selection will be taken as a justified selection.

8. Another important point to mention here is that what the interviewers have to do, they don't do, they do not want to do and they don't know how to do. Some unrelated questions about the cinema field, games field, etc., are occupying in the interviews. This type of questions in the interviews will show the ignorance and unable-ness of the interviewers. The interviewers must avoid such type of questions.

9. The interviewers should not think that whatever they knew are to be necessarily known to the candidates. It is a very bad thinking and practice on the part of the interviewers. One important fact is that the candidates also can ask questions from the Interviewers in the interview. Maximum Interviewers do not know this fact because they do not want to give a chance to the candidates. The candidates do not ask any questions in the interview because of the fear that they might not be selected in the interview, if they ask any question. Good interviewers must allow the candidate to speak more and create a situation so that the candidate may ask questions about the job for which he is attending the interview.

10. The interviewers should not give more importance for any questions on the subjects. Rather, the candidates are to be allowed to give a presentation on the matter of the choice of his own. The way of expression, management of time, method of teaching used by the candidates if it is for the post of teaching, way of his communication, and techniques of usage by the candidates are to be carefully noticed and judged. If it is administrative post, the different situations will be given to the candidate and he is to be asked how will he tackle the situation? How to control the students' unrest? Staff unrest? Environmental adverse conditions etc., are to be judged. All these judgments are to be done only after seeing the publications of articles and books.

11. The interviewers can go further, if they are fully satisfied with the candidate, the interviewers can carefully ask the questions like- " if you are given this post, what would be your concentrating areas to develop the institution?" The way in which the candidate submits his answer about the areas to be developed in the institution is to be carefully analysed and judged.
12. Each interviewer will award the marks for the candidates on the basis of the performance of the candidate. It should not be based on the group consultation of the interviewers inside the four walls. There is a possibility that the chairman of the interview board may influence the other members. Each interviewer's awards will be totaled, it will be added along with the Marks for publications, Books, Seminars etc, Marks obtained in the Qualifying Examinations etc. What is meant here is that there must be a formula to work out the selection. Interview alone should not be a criteria to select the candidate. What is that Criteria, Strategy , is to be decided well in advance.

Conclusion

So, Education is a unique feature that plays the most dominant role in the life and evaluation of mankind. A fully educated man is considered to be an important real human resource and hence, he is a tangible asset to the country. In fact, the economic growth and development of a country fully depends upon such real assets. Teachers, administrative officers, doctors, engineers, teachers, pilots, economists, scientists, writers, journalists, authors, workers, principals etc.,. are responsible for the Nation Building Project in the society. If they are good, every thing will be good and the vice versa is also true. There are excellent, dedicative, and hardworking people but at the same time there are few pathars (rice-less paddy) create hell of problems in every organisation. So right people are to be selected for the right job. Then only the expected results can be obtained and the goals can be achieved. It is the duty of the Interviewers to select the correct candidates by using a unpolluted systematic system and steps as is given above. The group is to be away from the influences of politics, drinks, money, and sex, etc., Once, if it is made and carefully implemented with the help of the dedicated persons, every office will have a real human asset and thereby quality of the work will be improved, cost of production will come down by increasing the efficiency and productivity and hence the Right Person will get Right Job in Right Time.

29

Concept of Science and Technology in the Economic Development

Present Scenario of Change

Our country has been coined as a developing country. In economics, developing countries were said to be under developed countries the development of a country fully depends upon the social, cultural, political and economic growth. Of all the above, the economic growth shares the maximum portion of the responsibility of development of a developing country and so the case of our country, India too. But the adverse growth of socio, cultural, and political aspects in the name of modernization and cut- throat will affect the overall development of the country even if there is a favourable growth in economic aspects. One can witness, the present scenario of dangerous social changes, terrible cultural explosions, and life killing political aspects, not only in one country, it is everywhere. So, to overcome such poisonous changes and to control such situation in the society, to safe guard the innocent young generation from such adverse change of socio, cultural and political aspects, there must be a strong, consistent economic development in the country.

Science and Technology

At the moment we say about the Science and Technology, the people started thinking it is something related to "the things" which can not be understood by every one. Of course only because of the science and technology, and the experts who have full knowledge about the science and technology, the business units of one country are able to attract and convert the consumers of the traders of the other countries as their (business units) customers. But it is not the case like that only certain people can understand about the science and technology. Anybody who really wants to know about or to become expert in science and technology can easily acquire the knowledge about the Science and Technology provided if he or she knows the concept of the Science and Technology well. As the people think, Science and Technology not only deal with high-tech business units but also deal with the following:

1. The advanced services,
2. Research and Development processes,
3. Creation of units,
4. Preparation of reports,
5. Creation of the effective and efficient managers,
6. Better utilisation of the human and non-human resources
7. Technology transfer technologies and
8. Purchase and sale of technologies
9. Innovation
10. Inventions,
11. New Ideas to solve the problems,
12. Product Planning, Product Designing,
13. Pricing,
14. Costing,
15. Accounting,
16. Management,
17. Marketing, also in
18. Motivating.

Science and Technology and Entrepreneurs

Now a days, the extent and scope of business of the business units do not confined to only internal and they go to competitive global level. For that, they have to find out a lot of new ideas and new products. This is not only for the profit making but also as a responsibility of the business units. So the entrepreneurs must have art and science of the business and the actives of the business and Management of the units. Innovation is the cover term for the activities of bringing new ideas and invention is the cover term for the activities of bringing something solidly in a physical shape to the world. Both invention and innovations are never ending process and path. The term entrepreneur means a businessman who has the qualities of inventions, innovations and risk bearing capacity. Industrialisation fully depends upon the qualities of the entrepreneurs of that country and the industrialisation is the base for the economic development of any country. The key factors for economic success are

Technology, Research and Development, and Knowledge Management, and most of all Innovation. Because the business units with the help of inventions and innovations become stronger, make more profits and generate more employment. To know the relationship of Economic Development and the of Science and Technology today, as is already told, one should understand the concept of "Economic Development & Industrialisation", "Economic Development & Science" and "Economic Development & Technology"

Economic Development and Industrialization

Economic development means the combination of economic growth and environmental protection. By keeping our environment under safe, the different sectors of a country namely, trade, commerce, industry, tourism etc. must grow to increase the per capita income, to increase the production, to increase the unemployment opportunities, to exploit the resources fully etc. This is possible only through industrialization. Industrialization is a sine – quo – none of the economic progress. All developed countries in the world are fully industrialized. Industrialization is one of the important means to improve the economy of the under developed. Industrialization is an effective instrument of growth and welfare. It gives the opportunity to any region to go for any international trade.

Requisite for Industrialization

Industry plays an important and vital role in the economic development. For this industrialization, Entrepreneurship quality oriented entrepreneurs are essentially required besides the other requirements of land, labour and capital. The entrepreneurship means the characteristics and quality of knowledge, art of carrying out, courage of facing the challenges, risk – bearing capacity, and art of making the product, and introducing the products in the market with marketing techniques. So, every entrepreneur should have the knowledge and art of doing business, which is, called science and technology.

Science and Economic Development

The term "Science" means "systematic body of knowledge". The economic development fully depends upon the industrialization, which has the basis of entrepreneurs with entrepreneurship qualities. So, the entrepreneurs are expected to have systematic body of knowledge about the business that they are going to do. They are expected to have thorough knowledge about the principles and functions of management, business, and all the activities related to the products. An entrepreneur particularly a scientific entrepreneur (not necessarily a science man) should always have thorough knowledge, systematic knowledge about the products, ingredients of the products, methods of productions, method of planning, organising and marketing the products. So, science plays a very vital role in the economic development.

Technology and Economic Development

Man started his race in different stages. Every stage is having its own importance and reasons for the closure. Succeeding stage came into existence with a new developed ideas and with the methods of usage and a lot of merits. He has made all his stages in his tools, clothing, fire, shelter, other survival items and even by making friendship with others. So the term technology is closely associated with advanced art of practice, submission and introduction. The term "technology" means "the systematic body of Mechanical and Industrial Arts". That means it is an art of mechanism and it is an art of industrial activities. Mere, having systematic body of knowledge done is not sufficient for an entrepreneur to become a successful industrialist to develop the economy. He is expected to have different arts of mechanism in the industry, different arts of production, art of innovations, art of inventions, art of marketing, art of controlling, art of communication, art of introducing a new product into the market etc. Then only the demand will increase, the production will increase, hence sales will go up and so on and the result will be the economic development.

Conclusion

Every businessman cannot be a successful businessman. The same manner, every inventor also cannot be a successful businessman. They are expected to know how to convert their technical work into economic performance and inventions into a business. This is possible only when the businessman/entrepreneur has the quality of science and technology. He should have thorough and systematic body of knowledge about business and he should also have the systematic body of knowledge mechanical and industrial business. Else, the other factors of production namely Land, Labour, Capital and Organization will become meaningless. So, science and technology is rightly ranked as the "fifth factor of production" which is the basis for industrialization, a base of Economic Development.

PART - IV

30

Problems Related Factors (P R F)

1. Corruption
2. Unemployment
3. Tax Reforms
4. Tsunami Problems

1. Corruption

1. Transparency is a Tool To Tackle Corruption

2. Unemployment

1. White Collared Unemployment
2. Planning a Suitable Career – A Professional Guidance
3. Management of Unemployment Problems
4. How To Conduct Interview?- A Model

3. Tax Reforms

1. Management of Tax Reform
2. Need For The Concept of Family Assessment in Tax Reform
3. Computation of Tax Liability of Co-Operative Societies

4. Tsunami Problems

1. Management of Post Tsunami Problems

31

Transparency is a Tool to Tackle Corruption

Abstract

In an exclusive definition, the corruption is defined as the "abuse of public office for private gain." It is a plague that attacks our society and economy as a whole. The corruption is the taste of the tasted cat. Now almost the corruption has become a common visible disease. It is very difficult to eradicate but can be tackled to maximum extent. The corruption will create harmful effects to the society. There are number of tools to tackle. Transparency is one of the efficient tools. By adopting the transparency techniques, the corruption can be tackled. Now the question arises – "What are to be transparented ?", "How to transparent" and "What are the preliminary works to be done"? The responsible persons must identify the Corruption Possible Centres (CPC), Affected Possible Persons (APP) and Possible Corrupt Persons (PCP). The applicant must know clearly about ways and means to get his dealings done through the concerned officers and employees without any fear and fever. Transparency of Persons, Transparency of Systems, Transparency of duties and responsibilities, Transparency of rights and powers, Transparency of requirements, Transparency of accountability, Transparency of accounts and audit reports, Transparency of punishments, Transparency of corruption, Transparency of awards and rewards, Transparency of action to be taken by superiors, and Transparency of redress are some of the methods of transparencies to tackle the corruption. Responsibility Accounting is to be introduced and it is to be managed effectively. A systematic Moral Education curriculum is to be drafted and the same is to be taught sincerely by the dedicated teachers.

Submission and Presentation

Corruption is like a virus to the computer, it is like a aids to the human kind. It will destroy each and every one of us at a particular stage. We can remove anything from us if others create it but we cannot remove the thing or behaviour from us if ourselves create it. So the Corruption is also like that it is very difficult to eradicate because we are creating the corruption. Every one of us knew what is corruption. We know that a man who is taking money to do his normal work is a corrupted person. Starting from the school admission, getting telephonic and electric connections, getting job, placing the paper on the table, till to see God's Dharshan in temple. We have to pay something more.

What is that Corruption?

In an exclusive definition, I can say that the corruption is defined as the "abuse of public office for private gain." It is a plague that attacks our society and economy as a whole. The corruption is the taste of the tasted cat. Once if it is tasted, then one cannot stop it and he will make everyone surrounding him to enjoy the taste to save his skin. This corruption is everywhere. But degree varies. At present, we can say as "he is less corrupted and the other is more corrupted. But the fact is that he is corrupted. To a normal layman, the following activities are corrupted activities:

(a) Taking huge money for the admission, for the appointments etc.
(b) Taking huge commission for the grant of tender only to a particular person.
(c) Taking huge share of such commission and putting the signature by the officer.
(d) Taking liquor and other intoxicants and helping a wrong and punishable culprit.
(e) Enjoying some facilities and granting some amenities.
(f) Helping a particular individual and delaying or not doing anything for another who is of same category.
(g) Taking money and giving result.
(h) Exercising the undue influences on the subordinates/relational persons.
(i) Going to the classes always late.
(j) Leaving the class students before the timings.
(k) Spending more time in taking attendance and talking irrelevancies inside the class.

(l) Wasting the time without doing the works to be done/carried out.
(m) Keeping the files without taking any action.
(n) Taking casual leave without producing leave/letter application.
(o) Taking wrong decision or a right case.
(p) Selecting a wrong person for the right job and vice versa by taking huge money.
(q) Taking more money and supporting the party men.
(r) Taking a favourable decision on a wrong case.
(s) Taking huge money and granting licenses.
(t) Taking huge money and granting contacts, international permissions etc. All are considered as corruption activities.

Even, the person who does no take money to do his normal work but becomes the reason for others taking money and the man who is causing such delay is also a corrupt man.

The corruption is divided into qualitative corruption and quantitative corruption. Qualitative corruptions are those activities of the corrupts and abuse of the public office for the private gain not in terms of money but in terms of the kinds/money – able values. Quantitative corruptions are those activities of the corrupts and abuse of the public office for the private gain in terms of money or cash. Of these two corruptions, though these two are dangerous, the qualitative corruptions are more dangerous.

Corruption is very dangerous to not only individuals but also Nation as a whole. Actually, it has to be eradicated completely. But the irresponsibilities of the responsible persons, mismanagement on the part of the managers, carelessness on the part of the officers, uncultured work culture of the workers and the employees have taken the corruption at present to an answerless question – whether the corruption can be eradicated completely? It has become a normal, now, like a diabetic disease which is almost become a domestic disease. Likewise, the corruption is everywhere and as diabetes cannot be eradicated completely but can be controlled, in the same manner corruption cannot be in short term totally eradicated but can be tackled, that is, controlled to some extent. There are many tools to tackle corruption. Of them transparency is one of the tools to tackle corruption.

By adopting the transparency techniques, the corruption can be tackled. Now the question arises – "What are to be transparented ?", "How to transparent" and "What are the preliminary works to be done"?

Transparency of Systems

Before establishing a business/work/project/ or any sequence of activities, the responsible persons must develop a systematic system. With internal check and internal control techniques, self – examinations and auto- detection of errors, mistakes, misrepresentation, undue influence and frauds. Such system will never allow any person to commit any ultra vires activities. The system is to be transpired and explained fully.

Transparency of Duties and Responsbilities

The duties and responsibilities are important ingredients of the Organisation. They are the factors responsible for the success of the main objectives of the Institution. These are the main centres where the corruption may try to enter. Everybody must be made known what they have to do and what they have not to do. If these duties and responsibilities of the individual officers, persons, employees, are made known to all the people or publicized i.e transparented, it is hopped that the corruption can be tackled.

Transparency of Rights and Powers

The Rights And Powers are another important ingredients of the Organisation. They are the factors responsible for the success of the individual employee or the officer in the Institution. These are the main centres where the individual allows the corruption to enter. Everybody must be made known what are their rights and what are their powers. If these rights and powers of the individual officers, persons, employees, are made known to all the people or publicized, i.e., transparented, it is hopped that the corruption can be tackled.

Transparency of Requirements

Another possible of the environment suitable to attract the corruption is the requirements required to get the things done through the government or from the government. The people are given the information about the requirements on piecemeal basis. They are called by the officers often to the counter. Such situation compels the applicant to compare the total cost involved and the corruption/ bribe to be given to get the things done through the particular officer. Once the requirements are made clear and are transparented, the applicant to some extent tackle the vicious circle of the corrupt officer.

Transparency of Accountability

In its democratic political aspect, decentralization as currently conceived and increasingly practiced in the international development community has two principal components: Participation And Accountability. Participation is chiefly concerned with increasing the role of citizens in choosing their local leaders and in telling those leaders what to do—in other words, providing inputs into local governance. Accountability constitutes the other side of the process; it is the degree to which local governments have to explain or justify what they have done or failed to do. Improved information about local needs and preferences is one of the theoretical advantages of decentralization, but there is no guarantee that leaders will actually act on these preferences unless they feel some sort of accountability to citizens. Local elections are the most common and powerful form of accountability, but other mechanisms such as citizen councils can have limited influence. The accountabilities are to be transparented. The elected bodies/leaders

Transparency of accounts and audit reports

Transparency of punishments

Transparency of corruption

Transparency of awards and rewards

Transparency of action to be taken by superiors

Transparency of redress

Steps to Control the Corruption

First, the responsible persons must identify the Corruption Possible Centres (CPC). Actually the Corruption Possible Centres are those areas in which or from which the possibilities of the corruption activities will start. An efficient officer or the manager can definitely find out the centres. The centres will differ from the office to office, organisation to organisation. The officer must always be vigilant on the Centres. Actually what is going at present, the responsible officer will never take any preliminary step to identify the cente. If he fails in identifying the CPC, the concerned officer can not control the corruption when it reaches the growing stage. Next, to identify Affected Possible Persons (APP) and Possible Corrupt Persons (PCP).

Advise to the Corrupt Persons

Please note that you are brought in by your Mother to this Holy land. You, the Corrupts are doing unexplainable, untolerable and inexpressible harm to your motherland. Again please note that you are the root cause of all evils, terrorism and loss of all moral values. You think that now you are very happy at the cost of morals and good souls. Don't forget that you are happily making both the Sin Provision and Sin Reserve for your Generation. Some times your generation may be good. Don't set aside their goodness and Happiness by your activity of corruption. Please change yourself, Try to make your souls immaculate and help in developing your motherland.

My Big Request

The Honorable administrators, the honorable university vice-chancellors, professors, Lecturers, teachers, scholars, lawyers, religious gurus, social workers, employees, who are having popularity, Fame, Drive, Dynamism in the country and whose policies and preaches are people-centered and human faced are being earnestly requested by my folded hands to constantly enliven the people for rooting out this evils of corruption by using your good offices for a healthy wealthy and a corrupt free society.

Conclusion

So in my conclusion, I wish to humbly submit that every one of us should sincerely fight against the corruption. Just now I told that one should get it in writing from the officer when he objects to do his normal work. It may be easy to say but in practice it is very difficult due to the accumulation of power and the unawareness of the related knowledge. At this juncture, we can not totally eradicate the corruption but we can control to some extent. The main reason is that we all have allowed the evil and devil through our leniency and less knowledge on the effective management without understanding the meaning and pain of the tears in the eyes of a dedicated and deserving persons. As a proverb goes, unless and until and if a thief himself is not changing from his base ideas, no one can change him. The situation is to be brought in the minds of every one that one should feel shame when he/she thinks about corruption.

32

White Collared Unemployment

Unemployment problem is one of our major problems. The number of unemployed people exceeds more than 25 millions. The live cards of job seekers in all Employment Exchanges in India are now around about 14 million. This includes Matriculates, Graduates but also Post Graduates and M. Phil holders. Out of many unemployment problems such as Agricultural unemployment problem and Industrial unemployment problem, seasonal unemployment problem, unemployment among educated population, which I want to refer here as White Collared Unemployment, is most dangerous disease for the peace and stability of a Nation.

Consequences

In India large number of people are completely jobless. Wherever they go they will have to see "No Vacancy" board. So this White Collared Unemployment leads to very tragic consequences. It breeds frustration in the minds of educated unemployed. The most serious aspect of the unemployment is the personal aspect. The man who is out of job may go through several stages of personal distress. First he suffers loss of income and whatever may be done to assist him, his whole outlook on life, and his decisions from day to day. In time he may also suffer loss of self-respect, with the growing conviction that he is unwanted and useless. Eventually, he may suffer loss of hope, and cease to care about finding a job. In a few cases of mental or emotional instability, unemployment is entirely a personal problem requiring personal treatment. Even somebody commits suicide. It has forced some of our talented Indian commercialists and management people, Engineers, and Doctors to migrate to foreign countries and to settle there permanently. Some of our educated youths because of frustration has become Naxalites. Our Ex-President Thiru V.V. Giri had rightly observed, as "Unemployment problem is the problem of problems Unemployment has made our youths Naxalites. Educated youths are deprived of all deserving comforts and their growing discontent has given scope for the speedy growth of Naxalism".

Causes

Many persons, including myself, are crying like anything about the unemployment problem particularly this White Collared Unemployment. Our Government, although is making many policies, should find the various causes and remedies for this unemployment among educated. Among many causes, here I want to give some causes.

Defective Education Formulae

Every year in India some new Universities and New Educational Institutions are being opened. Although it has been showing some developing signs, it is developing some dangerous problems of unemployment because of its ill functions. They are producing every year matriculates, Graduates, Diploma holders, Post graduates, M.Phil and Ph.D in terms of 000's. Almost the whole educational system is faraway from the object, which concerned with the practical facts of life. The graduates and Diploma holders and post graduates are feeded only with theoretical instructions. The Examination system in our India has been testing simply the mugging power of the students and the bookish knowledge of students accumulated over the years but not the intrinseque value intelligent i.e. mental acuteness and their creative processes. The traditional system of examination held at the end of the year encourages students to cram or to memorize what they learnt and how much they have been able to reproduce in the Examination hall within three hours. So crore and crore of our educated people who have no knowledge about truism of manual labour but by searching good jobs, are going without job.

Government's Reservation Policy

Our Government has been adopting a reservation policy for the past many years. Reservation of certain percentage of total number of jobs and Reservation of certain jobs and also fixing a special qualification to certain groups of population. Because of these Reservations and special qualifications the people, other than the people eligible for this reservation and special qualification are going without jobs even though they are fully and well qualified.

Character of Education

Yes, of course, no man can deny the fact that in our India the education is too literary which is away from the real life. But this much too literary education is not considered as fit for any job in present life. People, that's why, who has such education remain unemployed.

Huge Amount of Fees and Competitve Examinations

Almost now all sectors have started to adopt the recruitment procedure by conducting various tests. The fee, charges for the competitive examination is considerably more for example, for clerical Rs. 20 and for Probationary Officer test, Rs. 40 by BSRB. In rural areas, how an educated unemployed, whose father, who has disposed his only owned one-acre land for his son's education and is thinking what to do for tomorrow's rice, can pay Rs. 40/- as test fees, Rs. 3/- for typing the application form, Rs. 15 for passport photo ands Rs. 3.90/- for Registration charges. If the poor Post Graduate wants to apply, in his family all members / have to fast for 4 days. So these very qualified people are ill-fitted to participate as one of the candidate atleast of competitive examination and are going without job.

Political Parties Influences

Now we have been seeing many recommendations by the political Parties in all fields including education. The big authorities and Officers of various departments are compelled to do same work in favour of the person who gives recommendations through Political Leaders. So the right educated persons are not given the opportunity of getting jobs.

Defective System of Qualification Policy

Qualifications fixed by the Recruiting Authorities are irrelevant to the jobs concerned. The persons who have no knowledge about the Debit Entry and Credit Entry are recruited to the jobs which requires fully Debits and Credits. By doing so, this Debit and Credit Degree holders and going without job.

Disagreement between demand and supply of educated persons:-

Our Indian Universities and Education Institutions are producing unlimited matriculates. Graduates and Post Graduates if they just score 40%. But demand for these people is, of course, increasing but at a very slow rate. As a result of this the number of educated unemployed is increased year after year.

Lack of Industrial Development

Industrial development in our country is not only slow but also the regional distribution of Industries is exceedingly uneven and lacks scientific and technological base. The disproportionate growth of large scale Industries in a few areas gives employment opportunities for only the people who are living there. Other people particularly educated population living in a place where there is no industry such as Engineers, Technically trained and other Technocrats are going without jobs. A private industrialist prefers to continue with a low paid foreman rather than employed a qualified Engineer.

Female Competitions

Now-a-days the competition of female population has been increased in all fields. They are coming to all the fields including the field where in which the male population can only do. So as a consequence of their competition with male population for almost all jobs, our educated male population is going without jobs. This cause creates a dangerous frustration in the minds of educated males.

Suggestions

1. Education system must be overhauled completely at School and University levels. Instead of judging the students' knowledge in three hours of one year, should be judged atleast once in four months and average of those being declared as pass.
2. Semester system should be introduced in all Universities. Semester implies the division of the academic year into two periods. Semester system allows a higher degree of innovation and flexibility to students as well as teachers. As it has been widely used in advanced countries USA, USSR, Germany and Japan, in India also it has to be used fully.
3. Class room lecture should be reduced and that time must be utilized in supervised reading, Library work, Tutorials, Group discussions, Seminars, Problem solving and work assessment.
4. Apart from class room lectures there should be exposure of students to Industries and Factories, research laboratories, Social Service Organisations to enable them to acquire experience in the practical application of theoretical knowledge on the going project.
5. Recruitment procedure should be completely taken away. New suitable method must be introduced. In screening test and in interviews questions, which are related to job for which he is interviewed, must be asked.
6. The system, adopted by Government, of all pass upto VIII Std. Should be discarded. This education is just like bore less found less building. Primary school education is the foundation of Higher Studies. If he is just put from one Class to other Class without any foundation, he will struggle at his higher studies. So our Government should change this system.

7. The recruitment authorities should reduce the few of competition test and take the pearls in Rural oyster by giving the opportunities to educated unemployed who are in handicapped position to pay such huge fees.
8. Our Government of India must take steps to start various Industries at all places of our country and give the guidance as well as assistance to industries which are in dying position. Giving financial assistance and subsidy must encourage the Small Scale Industries and Cottage Industries. Of all this, the educated persons are to be encouraged to setup the self-employment, by giving proper training and financial assistance Which must be facilitated by removing all types of hindrances.

Education and recruitment should be separated as a separate sector, wherein which the prohibition must be made to all political influences. Our Government should relax the rules and regulations regarding the allocation of reservation policy. Our Government should take steps in these regards then only the right person can get right job.

33

Planning a Suitable Career -A Personnel Guidance

Introduction

Now a days, the expectation of students is that they should go for a best educational course which would give them excellent job opportunities, and to go for suitable jobs immediately after the completion of the school/college/university education. Also, it is the biggest problem of every parent to find suitable course or suitable job for their words after the formal education is over. Hence they are in need of career guidance. It may be easy to guide by any person to any person on any course/job. But all guidance may not be suitable to all the people. So, while guiding, the guide should necessarily think about the family background, health condition, the interests and habits, educational level, and the achievements of the candidate. Immediately after the completion of the school/college/university education, the parents and the students should think about his/her ward occupation, the future source for living. But one can not suddenly, then and there choose his/her career or occupation as and when they desire.

Career Guidance

Guidance carries the real message of education. It is not only a message for teachers and taught but also for parents. An individual needs guidance for many reasons like guidance for growth and development, guidance for creative thinking, guidance for problem solving, guidance for mental health, guidance for self-realization, guidance for healthy life, guidance to maintain equilibrium and for occupation/job. So, in real sense, guidance means an opinion, a point of view, or at best – a concrete suggestion which is never least mandatory that one may most earnestly request or others very graciously give one to analyse very rationally the alternate options available to him in his choices, plans, and adjustments to him in his choices, plans, and adjustments in life. Hence, Career Guidance, here, means an opinion, a point of view or a suggestion given by the author to the readers of the article.

So, before going to the higher education and immediately after the school education, the parents should meet the experts, the career guides (not a book but a person) with their wards. But most of us are not doing it. the parents and wards should clearly discuss their views, the family background, economic condition, wards' interest and wards' achievements etc. then the expert will properly advice. Some of the careers/services are given below as information:

Private Sector

Private occupation includes all positions starting from peon to the managing director appointed by the Private Sector. A good number of occupational opportunities to the youths to the less educated to the highly educated is provided by the private sector. Comparatively speaking in these days, this sector gives better salary and amenities than in government sector. To select occupation/employment in private sector any graduation/post graduation in the related area is sufficient.

Public sector

Generally, they are called "Corporations" in which the government will have substantial interest. Indian Airlines Corporation, LIC, NLC, IOC, ANIDCO, ANIFPCO are some of the examples of public sector undertakings. They provide a good number of employment opportunities to the candidates from less educated to the highly educated. Comparing with the private sector, this sector provides better job security.

Art and culture

In the present scenario "Art and Culture" is one of the sectors providing a lot of employment opportunities with attractive emoluments, benefits and publicity. It includes, drama, televisions, radio, cinema, painting, singing, etc. generally, it does not require any formal education. However, some big universities like Annamalai University have opened a separate college and institutions of Art and Culture. It is advised to the students that they have to practice themselves more.

Defence Service

Defence is another area which provides job opportunities to the young youths. Candidates who wish to serve Nation at the cost of their own lives are advised to choose this service. Defence provides variety of job opportunities like, defence doctor, defence engineer, defence teacher, soldier etc. For this purpose, one has to pass the relevant examinations like, NDA and other tests like physical fitness, mental alertness, ability etc. It is a respectful career. Qualification to enter into the defence service is from plus two to Doctorate depending upon the post for which the candidate applies.

Professional Service

The majority of the people are of the opinion that the professional service includes only Doctors and Engineers. But that situation has totally been changed in the present scenario. Professional service, now-a-days includes Income Tax Consultants, Business Consultants, Chartered Accountants, Cost Accountants, Career Guides, Doctors, Engineers, Advocates etc. They are independent people with particular expert knowledge. They enjoy respectful status in the society. People have good knowledge about the profession of Doctor and Engineer because now a days most of the unemployed youths are from these groups only. Surprisingly, the parents and the candidates have limited informative knowledge about the other professional services.

Personnel Service

This category includes all jobs under Civil Services namely IAS, IAAS, IPS, IFS, etc., and Banking, Railway, Audit, Postal, Income Tax, Judiciary and Excise etc. This personal services are considered high esteem by the people in the Society. It is believed that the best of human resources are being attracted towards this category. The students and candidates who have passed any degree are eligible to appear for the civil service examinations. Due to the highness of the category, now-a-days, even the persons the highest qualifications like Ph.D and D. Lit and higher qualifications of M.Com, MBA, MCA etc also started entering into this service.

Teaching service

The most divine and highly respected service is the teaching service. The teachers are highly valued and respected by the society because they are the bases of the Nation. For the Teaching Service, a bachelor/master degree in the concerned subject with a degree or diploma in education is required depending upon the class for which the candidates are to be recruited.

Self - Engaged Occupation

People are of the view that self-employment is a last resort to the people who could not get jobs/ employment/occupation in private, public, cooperative, art and music, government sectors. But, it is not the fact. Self-occupation is not only providing employment to the person concerned but also makes provision for others. Business, tourism and travels, industrial units, commercial units, fisheries, poultry, piggery is the area in which one can think about for the self-employment. It is considered to be best because, it helps the economy in many ways by removing unemployment problem, by contributing tax and savings. It does not require qualifications but practical knowledge. Business includes all industrial, commercial and trade activities. Doing business at this present economic conditions require a lot of knowledge and tactfulness. But it is an excellent service area. Production and Supply of goods and services to the needy consumers and customers to their fullest satisfaction is just an un-measurable and un-scalable ethical aspect. If one starts business activity, the governments do give a lot of concessions, subsidies and bounties. He need not have to worry about his own employment/job and also he can give job opportunities to the young and educated youths, and by doing so, he can enjoy a status of an employer. Since the government can not provide employment opportunities to all the educated youths, the present need is to start his/her own business unit. For business, it is advised to go for a B.Com, BBA, BCS, BA (Eco) etc. courses.

Present Status

Now-a-days there is a heavy demand for the degrees related to Business Education such as B.Com, BBA, BCS, M.Com. MBA, MCA, MFM, ICA, ICWA, ICS, CFA, etc., compared with the other courses. Equally other personal services like IAS, IPS, IAAS, IRS etc., too have heavy demand. To become a Chartered Accountant (CA), one has to pass examination conducted by the Institute of Chartered Accountant of India. Minimum qualification is passed plus two. There are three stages namely foundation, inter and final. All papers are commerce based with mathematics and law. Likewise the Cost Accountant and Company Secretary also have the same positions. Any intelligent student can very easily pass ICA, ICWA, ICS Examinations. Master of Business Administration (MBA), Master of Financial Management (MFM), Master of Computer Applications (MCA), Master of Commerce (M.Com) and High Status Diplomas like Personnel Management and Industrial Relations etc., are best courses for the excellent profession.

Suggestions

My dear readers, I hope, you might have understood the various classification to the careers/jobs, the related qualifications and their status and importance from the above discussion. My dear young friends and respected parents, I have given few suggestions to choose your career.

1. Do not insist your son & daughters (wards) to go for any particular course/job.
2. Carefully watch the area of interest in your wards.
3. Till your wards reach the 10th Standard/Class, do not wash his/her brain with any suggestions. After reaching 10th Standard, the parents, should start telling him about the family background, family financial position, employment opportunities, merits and demerits of the various occupations, his area of interests, etc.
4. When he or she completes the 10th Standard, please meet a career expert with your ward. Clearly explain the expert what is mentioned above (in Point No. 4) and discuss open heartedly with your wards.
5. Allow your wards to talk and raise questions with the Career Expert.
6. Do not come to a conclusion with the career expert in one visit.
7. Choose atleast three alternative course of actions.
8. Go home and discuss with his/her mother, brother as you have discussed with the expert. Compare the advantages and disadvantages with your financial conditions and other loan facilities.
9. Choose a particular course and concentrate fully upon the course without giving any room for confusion.

Conclusion

Once the parents and wards collectively take decision after meeting the Career Expert by analyzing the different variables, determinants, factors, etc., I hope that a right person will go for right job. Hence a valuable Human Resource may be created, productivity will be increased; and I am sure that the economic development of our country will be increased in Real Term.

34

Management of Unemployment Problems

Introduction

Unemployment is the real problem of a country. It is a social problem. It is very dangerous than the Poison. It is just like an acid thrown skin to the development of the Nation. It is a great threat to the country and its development. It creates inequalities of income, economic imbalance and frustration in the minds of the young educated youth who are going to be the tomorrow's administrators. Unemployment Problem is like a gnat which gnaw away and sift away the concentration of the administrators on the development of the country. The unemployment problem kills the family as a whole. It tempts the unemployed youths to commit suicides for the want of every day's bread and social prestige. Due to this unemployment problem, the youngsters will be attracted towards the unwanted and anti-national elements. The unemployment problem is a great obstacle to the economic growth. If it is not properly managed or even if it is lightly taken the country will face terrible problems. The unemployed population will become a untolerable problem and heavy chronic disease to the country. Mere introducing some schemes which will work for some temporary time, as we show some toys to the crying child, will definitely not solve the purpose. There must be a constructive policy, strategy, rules, procedures besides the planning to save the country from the explosion of the unemployment problem. This is to be managed very carefully which is the need of this hour.

Management

Generally the term Management refers, "getting things done through others by going with others". Analysation of the above quotation gives us a lot of meanings that all works are to be done in right way, in right time, in right combination and in right relations. The management is really an art. Everyone can not do it satisfactorily. The main reason for the slow economic growth is only the majority of the organisations, units, institutions, departments, sections, offices, etc. are managed by the people who have less qualities of such art. It is quiet natural that if a driver without knowing driving drives a truck, it will definitely meet with accident by taking the lives of the many people and truck itself will be no more. If a teacher with out teaching qualities and capacities is appointed, he will certainly destroy the future of the innocent students who are the future of the country and the country as well. Hence, the management plays a very vital role in the every field and so it is very essential in the never ending and slow killing unemployment problems. It is not that much difficult how it is presently being thought of if it is properly managed with positive attitudes. The management of unemployment problem consists the following:

1. Understanding the Present Scenario
2. Understanding the Principles
3. Functions of Management
4. Management of Suggestions

Present Senario

Everybody knows about the problem of unemployment. Everybody starting from the Academicians to Politicians including the Government talk about the unemployment problems. But the outcome of such talks is nil. Everybody would like to get job as early as possible through one way or other. Bribing, Recommendations Pressure through Politicians and Rulers, Undue Influence, Misrepresentations, Coercion and Fraud are also the ways through which the people get employment. Something are known and some other things are not known. Another point to be taken for the high level thinking is that the manner, velocity and the position of the employment actually prevailing in India at present. We have been witnessing that in one family (FI), husband, wife, sons, daughters, daughter-in-laws etc. all are employed but at the same time in some families (FII) nobody even husband or wife or son will not get even 0.5 employment. It is not untrue. In fact it is what actually going in our country.

If one starts thinking, analysing and interpreting the cause and situations, the answer we will get is that our country do not have the employment policy. One more point we have to note here is that in the present scenario, the people think that the main purpose of taking degree is to go only for job as their primary option and for the knowledge etc. are only the secondary options. Of course, the population supporting the FI group will never accept rationale employment and the population supporting the FII group will always oppose the FI Group. The others will always support for the rationale employment. At the present scenario of political set up, administrative set up the activities of these groups are like rat and cat game and the result will be the Unemployment Problems affecting economic growth like a slow killing poison.

The life of the family belongs to the FI Group will be flourishing due to the principles of comparative advantages. The savings, investments, tax concessions, more chances to escape from the tax liabilities, position in the society, medical facilities, allied advantages to get favoritism, returns from the investments and savings, purchase of the wealth etc. are the enjoyments and sophisticatedness of the FI Group Family. Whereas the Family belongs to FII Group for the want of unemployment even for 0.5 employment first starve, next they will not have better cloths, and it is quiet natural they can not go for food even for half stomach every day. They might have sold all their properties for the education expecting that they will get opportunity of getting jobs. Then the questions related to the enjoyments and sophisticatedness do not arise and they can not even think about all such factors, it will become almost fiction in their lives and finally they will have to go for decisions and thinking like going away from the universe or they will be attracted by some anti-social animals.

Principles of Unemployment

Actually the term principle means the fundamental truth as such the Principles of Unemployment means the fundamental truth of the Unemployment. Before solving the problem or taking any measure to solve the problem, one should understand clearly the fundamental reason for and truth of the problem and there should be no compromise in understanding the problem. Any suggestion, solution or any attempt to take corrective steps of any issue or any problem irrespective of the size will certainly go waste if the principles are not properly understood. As such, even in our country many projects and systems fail continuously. Unemployment is a situation that arises when a particular factor does not find place for its role for economic return. Of the factors of production- land, labour, capital and organisation- labour is the only factor has Natural Life and has the capacity to express its pain when it is not finding place for its economic role for its source of income. The other factors are mixed by the human factor in the process of production and business.

Hence, the unemployment is a common term applicable for the factors of production. If any one of the factors of production is unemployed, the society, the government, the population etc. will have the adverse impact and will be affected very badly. The productivity of that particular unemployed factor will be zero and that will be continuously affecting the productivity of the other factors of production. Here, the unemployment of the labour factor i.e-human factor is being taken in this piece of work. The principles of the human unemployment factor are having cause root of the increasing nature in geometric progression with no corresponding increase in the subsistence. The responsibility is with everybody to put a check for the growing population. In a general and normal condition, it can not be managed.

Another reason for the unemployment of human factor is the want of Nature's Support. Here also, the human force can not manage the Nature's Role. Such unemployment is called seasonal unemployment. This will be in the agricultural sector. The best example is the states are fighting for the water and due to the non-availability of water, the acute unemployment problem in the agricultural sector of the respective states. There is one more reason for the unemployment is that the change in the market (of all kinds) situation. That is the cyclical nature of the business in the boom and depressions. This unemployment is completely in the Business Sector. Though this reason can be thought of for the control but practically, now-a-days, it can not be managed. One more dangerous reason for unemployment is the dissatisfied employment and non-availability of job for the educated human force. This is called disguised unemployment. This is very dangerous because the productivity of such dissatisfied employee will be zero and even it will go to minus.

Principles of Pro-Rata

If the articles are more, the question does not arise how much is to be given to people per head. The people can be allowed take as much as they want. But if the heads are more than the available articles, then one has to seriously think about the sharing of the available articles. The same manner, if the employment opportunities are more, then it can be given to all people irrespective of the restrictions. But the employment opportunities are less than the eligible and qualified people, then the problems of unemployment will arise and hence the question of the management of the employment and the unemployment problem will arise. By carefully managing, the qualified people are to be given the jobs and at the same time it should be proportionately given to the eligible and qualified candidates in such a way that at least one in a family will get a job. This is called principles of pro-rata.

Functions

The following are the essential functions of the Management of Unemployment Problems:

1. Effective Planning with Procedures, Rules, Strategics and Policies.
2. Careful Organising with Authorities, Responsibilities, Delegation & Decentralization.
3. Clear-cut Communication with the necessary directives and directions
4. Powerful Controlling with Feed-Back Techniques and
5. Sensible Coordination

Effective Planning

As far as the employment in our country is concerned, the planning is not effective and one can take that it is almost nil. Planning means "What to do? What not to do? How to do? and Who will do?" To remove the unemployment problem though not 100 % atleast to some extent, the government should plan effectively through the experts and dedicated persons who knew the matters. Policies, Rules, Procedures and Strategies are to be carefully drawn. Carelessness in framing the policies and rules etc., will again bring the present situation.

Careful Organising

After having drafted the effective planning, they are to be carefully organised with the qualified personnel. Yes Masters, Chair Parasites, Power Wanties, Drinkers, Office Politicians, etc., are to be totally avoided while selecting the qualified personnel for the proposed careful organising. They must be dedicated towards the job and loyal to the career. They are to be work cultured. Organising means the method by which the men and materials are combined to achieve the desired goals. Here the desired goal is to remove the unemployment problems. The proposed organising must carefully take over the activities as per the planning and execute the same with authorities and responsibilities, through the delegation and decentralization.

Clear-Cut Communication

Communication is the nervous system of the organisation. In today's scenario, a lot of unproductive payments are being made due to the want of clear-cut communication. After committing the mistake, the people tactfully escape by telling the word " it is the communication gap". Since the suggestions given in this piece of work are the forecasting of the actual happenings in near future, information are to be reached and received. By adopting the downward and upward and horizontal methods, the communications are to be given and obtained. The policies, rules, procedures etc., prepared in relation to the management of the unemployment problems are to be made familiar and crystal clear among the people at large.

Control

Control is the monitoring activity in the process of management. Control-less management is like a brakeless running vehicle. Management of unemployment problems requires more control and effective feed back system. The responsible officers in the process of management must compare the standard i.e what should have happened as per the policy, rules and procedures etc., of the new employment system and what has actually happened in the various stages of implementing the above policies etc.. this is to find out the favourable changes and adverse changes while implementing the managerial activities of removing the unemployment problems.

Coordination

The whole process of management of unemployment problem will go waste and failure if the sensible coordination is not there. Generally coordination means orderly arrangement of group effort for common purpose. Here in this context of the management of unemployment problems, the sensible coordination means the activities of bringing the principles, management of suggestions, present scenario, and the orderly arrangement of group efforts of the employer, government, and the unemployed youths/persons to achieve the balanced economic development in our country. The people who are responsible for such coordination have to be very careful while coordinating the group efforts. Of course, this is not an easy work because, the work is to be performed by getting criticisms from majority of the people.

Management of Suggestions

To manage the problems of unemployment means, creation of employment opportunities in a very balanced way. Principles of unemployment, Principles of pro-rata, Present scenario etc., are to be very carefully understood without any selfish and negative attitude. Positive thinkings are the vitamins and minerals of the body of the management of unemployment problem. A man or a group of men without positive thinking and with out the knowledge of the Principles of unemployment, pro-rata and the present scenario can not manage the unemployment problems. Effective Planning, Careful Organising, Clear-cut Communication, and

Tactful Coordination are to be practiced by the personnel who are going to be placed in the process of management of unemployment. The following measures are suggested.

1. In the present day situation, one can not simply say that one sex is superior or inferior to the other sex. Cent per cent both female and male are to be treated equally and that is the Nature's Law also. In a family, the husband and wife should never think that one is superior and other is inferior hence control can be exercised on other. Both Husband and Wife must feel that they are made for each other, they are equal in rights, having equal responsibilities and duties, sharing equally the liabilities etc. If it is the case, then the family will be a happy home. The children will come up without any shortfalls. The same manner, every family must think about the welfare of the Nation also. Welfare of the Nation means the welfare of the families. Nation can not be in a state of Welfare when there is an imbalance among the families within the available resources. So it is suggested to have a policy of One Family One Employment. Here the family means Husband, Wife, Children of age below 21 years (unmarried daughters till their marriage). Home management is equally important to the earning by going outside on job/employment. Let the members of the family decide who will go for job and who will manage the home. People under FI group may criticise for this suggestion. But this is the fact that one day or other we will be forced to make this suggestion as the employment policy.

2. At present the Retirement Age is fixed at 58 years to 60 years and in some cases it is even upto 62 years. The retirement age as above was fixed when the country faced the problems of employment, when there was dearth of educated qualified personnel, when there was no commerce, management, accounts and specialised courses and experts, when the population was limited and in a controllable stage and when there was no unemployment problem. But now the situation is totally reverse. Plenty of specialised experts are available in the employment market. The employers started bargaining with the candidates for employment. Now a days, well qualified candidates performed to work even at low salary. Considering the welfare of the Nation, more availability of well qualified candidates, the pathetic conditions of the educated well qualified unemployed youths, the decreasing marginal productivity of the aged employees, it is suggested to reduce the age limit for the Retirement to 55 years with immediate effect and 54 years after 5 years, 53 after 10 years, 52 years

after 15years, 51 years after 20 years and 50 years after 25 years from the current year.

3. Giving special concessions to a particular group of employees is to be stopped immediately. Taking care of children is to be considered as very important. This is not only at the interest of the particular family but also at the interest of the Nation as a whole since today's children are the tomorrows Leaders, Scientists, Doctors, Engineers, Educationists, Accountants, Managers and Administrators etc. In a nutshell they are the real Human Assets of the country. So it is suggested that government must take steps to take care of the children through any one of the parents. The necessary Rules are to be made. Any one of the parents will go for job and other one will take care of children since they are the human resources of our country. The parents may decide who will go for job and who will take care of their children.

4. To avoid the problems of unemployment, necessary awareness is to be brought in the minds of the people particularly in the minds of the educated young youths about the possibilities of starting of the self employment, available resources, available assistance like subsidies, concessions, bounties etc., In fact they do not know about all these things. It is understood from a survey among the educated unemployed youths. The government must come forward to help them by extending their helping hands through the governmental departments without terrorize them by telling complex rules and regulations. Hence, it is suggested to give a meaningful training to the concerned staff on " how to treat and encourage the young entrepreneurs" . Due to delay on the part of the govt. agencies, many entrepreneurs have lost their full strength of starting any unit. Necessary meaningful training is to be given to the new entrepreneurs on the trade concerned for the considerable period.

5. The views and thoughts of the government employees on the "concept of government employment" and the extent of their feeling about the government employment is to be understood properly by them. They should realise that the government is giving so much of facilities to them for the purpose of increasing their productivity and not for the purpose of criticizing others without doing job and without the having the principles of esprit de corps. A strict system is to be made in every govt. offices so that the employees must feel that they have to work with increasing productivity. The true meaning

of the term human relations is to be understood by all the employees in a very right way. Human relations are important but it doesn't mean that the workers and employees are to be satisfied always by cutting their productivity. Everybody must proud to say that they are working in government sincerely. Hence it is suggested to have a system in every offices in such a way if any employee is not contributing or the productivity is coming down or declining day by day or creating huge trouble to the normal atmosphere, they are to be removed by doing all legal formalities. In their place, other qualified persons are to be appointed immediately.

6. No one can deny the fact that we face Unemployment Problem. If any employee whether he is government servant or non government servant would like to go for employment in abroad on contract basis for one or more years or on permanent basis, it is suggested that immediately the related controlling officers should encourage and allow him to go abroad by sanctioning the necessary leave. The officer who leaves for abroad is to be made very clear that he would be given retirement benefits only for the period worked in our country. And in his place one or two people under divisible salary system are to be appointed. For example, one employee with a monthly salary of Rs. 30,000 wishes to go for abroad on a contract basis for period of 5 years. Immediately he should be encouraged to go by granting leave for a period of five years with a option to extend the leave for a period of another five years. In his place 6 persons and that too fully qualified persons can be employed at a monthly salary of Rs. 5000 each or atleast 03 persons @ Rs. 10000 can be appointed for ten years. Hence, it is suggested to have separate rules for such cases. 50% of the problems will be solved if this suggestion is seriously implemented through the dedicated personnel. But some places due to the adamant nature, the officers create hell of problems not only for the employee who wish to go abroad but also to the country as well by objecting remarking and rejecting the proposals by thinking they have power to do so.

7. At present, the government faces a lot of crises in the management, finance, less productivity and problems due to unemployment. Pension and Gratuity are being paid to the government employees. But the private sector employees generally do not get pension and gratuity equal to the government employees. Moreover, the activities and attitudes of the government employees as far as the productivity is concerned has been concerning the government and force to go

for privatization. Hence it is suggested to stop the pension and gratuity for the newly recruited employee through a suitable revised salary structure. Let them plan for their old aged savings schemes. Now a days, plenty of savings schemes are available both in the government sector and in corporate sector.

8. As on today some would like to retire from the service at the early age i.e at the completion of their 10th, or 15th, 20th year from their date of initial appointment. But the government puts some rules and regulations that one can retire only at the completion of 20th year. When this rule was originally made, it was correct due to that situation. But now the situation is entirely changed. The country has been facing untollerable unemployment problems and other problems due to the unemployment problems. So it is suggested to implement the suitable schemes so that the employees can go for voluntary retirement even at the completion of their 10 year onwards by taking the above suggestion.

9. At present, the Employment Exchanges function maximum for the government sector. The private sector selects their employees with out any general system and common procedure. They adopt their own procedures. Hence it is suggested that the Private Sector should also select the people/employees only through the employment exchanges. Also it is suggested that the necessary instructions may be given to the employment exchanges.

10. Another important problem is that the young unemployed youths do not have enough guidance. They feel that they are not taken care of by the governments. They even don't know about the available resources in their area, and other facilities available to start the ventures. So it is suggested that the government must order and accelerate the activities of the District Industries Centres (DIC) to go for the detailed study for the resources available in the particular district with its real economic viabilities and feasibilities. Table study techniques are to be totally avoided. This will be ending in the unproductive payment of salaries. Hence it is suggested a real economic survey on the feasibilities and viabilities of the various projects for the self employment within the resources available locally is to be conducted. The survey must be based the real figures and the same should be conducted sincerely and seriously. The government may direct the concerned offices to take expert opinions and even some guidance like special lectures, group discussions, meeting with special points, etc., from the locally available commerce

professors particularly who have done research works on the industries.

11. It is also suggested that the above surveys are to be made available to the educated unemployed youths. The concerned authorities must advertise and publicize in such a way that the unemployed should come forward to start the self employment through industrial and commercial ventures. A one hour duration documentary film is to be produced covering the resource availability, scope of opening the industrial ventures, available concessions, subsidies, bounties etc., government support, provisions for the space in the industrial estate, loan facilities, to whom one should go and approach etc., and the same film is to be screened in the important places like colleges and universities.

12. Where is will there is a way. Now a days number of universities have introduced the Distance Education Programmes covering almost all the curriculums. To have their management network, they approach the existing educational institutions and handover the full charge of managing the affairs related to the teaching, contact programmes, correction of assignments, conducting practicals. Conducting examinations etc., The universities appoint coordinators, asst coordinators, counselors, clerks, typists, waterman, call boys, peons, messengers, etc., They provide funds for the separate newspapers, magazines, journals, books etc. All the above persons are appointed from the existing employees of the institutions. They earn multiple income in multiple ways. For example, a senior lecturer is appointed as Coordinator or Asst. Coordinator in a Distance Education Programme. In his capacity of Senior lecturer he earns around Rs. 30,000 pm. In the capacity of Asst. Coordinator or Coordinator he earns Rs. 1,500 pm, Then he earns Rs. 2400 pm for counseling the classes @ Rs. 300 per class for two classes every Sunday. In addition he earns on an average Rs. 1,500 pm in the name of assignment correction and Rs. 2000 to 3000 as the Superintendent by enjoying the office benefits. Let them earn, that is not a question. Every teacher is given a minimum period and maximum period to teach. The principle of the maximum and minimum periods of teaching is that every teacher needs maximum rest so that they can contribute more to the students by preparation of latest knowledge. If they are sitting and spending more time in other activities, definitely they can not contribute more time to teach. They will try to skip their normal work for which they are originally appointed.

Conclusion

So, the unemployment problems are the dangerous challenge for the development of and the chronic disease to the country. All are not responsible for such disease. There are best officers, administrators and politicians in our country. But their views and ways are not taken over and are not given much weightage and importance. So the policies are made, rules are framed with the valuable view of such best people. This is resulted in the unemployment, become the unemployment problems, growing to the extent of barriers to the development and in due course the problem become the irremovable barriers and incurable disease of the Nation. If an effective strategy is framed in the light of the above discussion and suggestions, it is certainly believed that the unemployment problems will be solved and everybody will be happy and enjoy the taste of the life, real human resources may be created, youngsters will have confidence in their lives, the education will definitely will have real meanings, imbalances will be totally removed and the right person will get right job through the balanced way Hence, the country will be economically developed.

(Please see a diagram below)

MANAGEMENT OF UNEMPLOYMENT PROBLMES

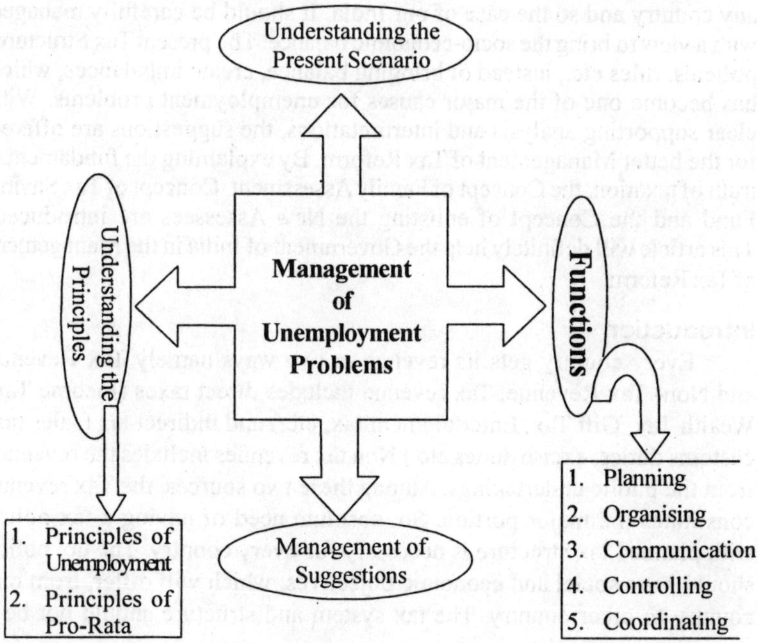

35

Management of Tax Reform in the Economic Growth

Abstract

India is a paradox in many ways. It is Blessed with a lot of Natural Resources including Manpower. But due to the lack of efficient management of the different sectors and absence of clear-cut policies, procedures, strategies etc., India is still in developing stage with the chronic problems like poverty, unemployment, illiteracy, social and economic imbalances etc.. Tax Revenue constitute the major portion of income to any country and so the case of our India. It should be carefully managed with a view to bring the socio-economic balance. The present Tax Structure, policies, rules etc., instead of bringing balance, create imbalances, which has become one of the major causes for unemployment problems. With clear supporting analysis and interpretations, the suggestions are offered for the better Management of Tax Reform. By explaining the fundamental truth of taxation, the Concept of Family Assessment, Concept of Tax Saving Fund and the Concept of enlisting the New Assessees are introduced. This article will definitely help the Government of India in the Management of Tax Reform.

Introduction

Every country gets its revenue in two ways namely Tax Revenue and Non- Tax Revenue. Tax revenue includes direct taxes (Income Tax, Wealth Tax, Gift Tax, Entertainment tax, etc.) and indirect tax (sales tax, customs duties, excise duties etc.) Non tax revenues includes the revenues from the public undertakings. Among these two sources, the Tax revenue constitutes the major portion. So, absolute need of having a tax policy with planned tax structure is necessary for every country. The tax policy should have social and economic objectives, which will differ, from one country to other country. The tax system and structure should not be a mere speed walk in the dark. So, depending upon the economic situation prevailing in the country, the tax system, structure and policy are to be constructed. If any tax system already exists, then it should be carefully managed with a view to bring socio economic balance. In the process of management, new concepts are to be brought in by giving more importance to the principles of taxation and , social & economic objectives. This process is called Tax Reform. The present piece of work concentrates upon the management of the reform in the present scenario of our country with special reference to the individual taxpayers particularly the salaried group.. Discussions and measures given in this paper are only suggestions. Accepting or rejecting is absolutely in the hands of the learned people and the government.

Management of Tax Reform

Our country is a developing country. Everyone knows that the economic growth in our country is very slow and it is to be accelerated. There are many reasons like unemployment problem, social inequalities, under-exploitation of the resources and the slow growth of savings and investments for such slow growth.. In the absence of suitable tax policy, and the tax structure, the rate of economic growth will be sluggish. So the tax reform is the answer for the above problem and it is to be managed very carefully with the

Management of Tax Reform

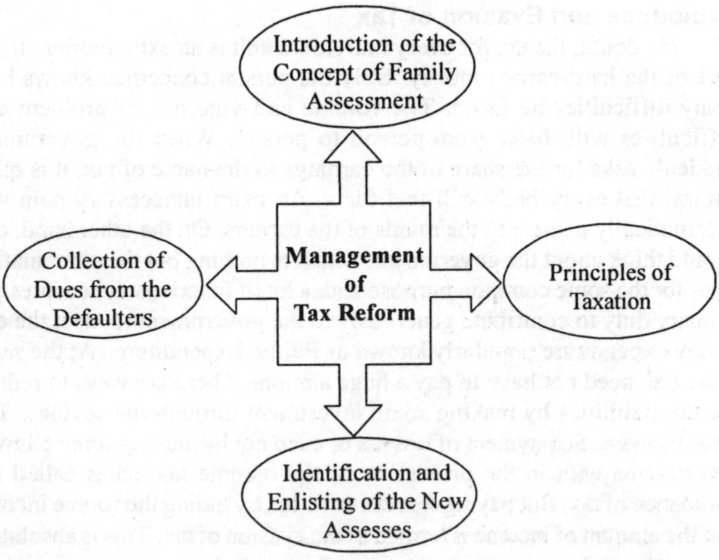

Fig. 01

principles of taxation, introduction of the new concepts by encouraging the savings and investments. The following are the ingredients of the management of Tax Reform.

1. Understanding the Income Tax
2. Avoidance and Evasion of Tax
3. Changes made by the Finance Bill 2003
4. Present Scenario
5. Principles of the Taxation
6. Understanding Standard Deduction
7. Understanding Savings & Investments
8. Introduction of the New Concepts
9. Identification and Enlisting the New Assess
10. Collection of Dues from the Defaulters

Income Tax

Tax, Levy, Toll, Duties, etc give the same meaning. But they differ from the purposive income and situation on which it is calculated. All are the compulsory payments to be made to government or to the persons authorised by the government. Hence tax is the compulsory payment to be made to the government. As such the Income Tax means the compulsory payments to be made to the government based on the income of the person calculated as per the provisions of the Income Tax Act.

Avoidance and Evasion of Tax

No doubt, the tax for every individual/unit is an extra burden. It is a part of the hard-earned money. Only the person concerned knows how many difficulties he faced. The volume and vigorous of problem and difficulties will differ from person to person. When the government suddenly asks for the share of the earnings in the name of tax, it is quite natural that every body will feel for it. An extra unnecessary pain will automatically come into the minds of the earners. On the other hand, one should think about the government, which is nothing but the combination of us for the some common purpose with a lot of functions. It becomes our primary duty to contribute generously to the government to meet the day to day expenditure popularly known as Public Expenditure.. At the same time, one need not have to pay a huge amount. There are ways to reduce the tax liabilities by making some investment through the savings. The Law allows it. So payment of less tax or even not by making some allowed investments with in the provisions of the income tax act is called the avoidance of tax. But paying less tax or no tax by hiding the source income and the amount of income is termed as the evasion of tax. This is absolutely against the Rule and will attract a lot of complications even upto court.

Changes brought by the Finance Bill 2002 & Finance Bill 2003

It is the normal practice of the Govt. Of India to bring changes in the Taxation through the Finance Bill of that year. As such the Govt. of India passed the Finance Bill in the year 2002 i.e Feb 2002, which has made a large number of significant, changes in the taxation of individuals. The maximum tax free limit for the individuals i.e. the basic limit and the rates of income tax for each slab are not changed. Hence the maximum tax free limit is only Rs. 50,000. As far as the rates are concerned, it is 10% from Rs. 50001 to Rs. 60000., 20% from Rs. 60001 to Rs150000 and 30% for income beyond Rs. 150000. But the Finance Bill brought an additional liability of 5% surcharge (tax on tax). Till last year 20% rebate on tax was given on the eligible savings subject to the limitation of Rs. 12,000 whereas for the Assessment Year 2003-04 the rebate on tax is reduced to 15% with a nominal increase in the limitation of savings i.e from Rs. 60,000 +Rs. 20,000 = Rs. 80,000 to Rs. 70,000 + Rs. 30,000 = Rs. 1,00,000. However, the individuals whose income after the Standard Deduction (SD) is upto Rs. 1,50,000 the rebate is allowed at the rate of 20%. But the individuals whose income after the SD is more than Rs. 5,00,000, he is not entitled for any rebate. Deduction for interest on housing loan can be claimed upto Rs. 1,50,000. These are some of the changes brought by the Finance Bill 2002 as far as the individual taxpayers (salaried group) is concerned.

The Hon'ble Finance Minister Shri Jaswant Singh in the parliament presented the Union Budget 2003-04 on 28th Feb., 2003. The important changes brought in are that the standard deduction limit has been raised from Rs 25,000 to 40% or Rs 30,000, whichever is less for those earning below Rs 5 lakh per annum,. But if the annual salary is over Rs 5 lakh, then the standard deduction limit will be Rs 20,000 only. The 5% surcharge levied in last budget has been removed for individuals. The total deduction of Rs 9,000 earlier available under section 80L with regard to income from dividend and interest has been upped to Rs 12,000. Interest rate on investment in PPF and small savings has been further reduced by 1% from March 2003. Indian citizens have to compulsorily furnish PAN numbers for foreign travel. Procedures and methods for search and seizure operations during income tax survey have been simplified and individual taxpayers have to fill single-page income-tax return form for filing IT returns

Present Scenario

Every Individual taxpayer anxiously waiting for the day of the budget presentation by the Hon'ble Finance Minister in the Lok Shabha. They are very keen to note the points favourably that are being announced. The cute and ambitions are more in case of the salaried group of people among the individuals taxpayers. All individuals particularly the salaried group seriously think that there is no much change in the tax structure for the past few years. The government has reduced the rate of interest on the different types of deposits and savings. This discourages the individuals to go for the savings in the regulated market. As the result, the private circulation has started flourishing. Chit Funds, Yela Cheetu, Finance for Kenthu Interest, private money lending, lump sum money lending, leasing finance etc., started coming up. Of course, in the long run, no doubt, the people have to go to the regulated markets for their savings. It is not that much clear why the government has reduced the interest rates on the savings. The government could have earned more out of the differential rate of interest without reducing the rates. A detail is given in the suggestions. The female taxpayers are given extra incentives of tax concession ie., upto Rs. 5000 which is equal to Rs. 5000x100/20= Rs. 25000 savings. Some of the taxpayers feel that this facilities may be extended to all.

Now a number of talks are going in the name of tax reforms to remove the Standard Deduction, removal of considering the accrued interest on the house building advance, removal and reduction of the tax rebate system, changes in the rates of income tax etc. One side the government does not want the present rate of interests another side the government wants to forgo the considerable amount of savings by discriminating the employees by sex. This is nothing but the loss of revenue to the government. Here the hidden principle, for such reduction of rate of interest, giving special concessions, discriminating the employees by sex, forgoing the considerable amount of savings, indirect encouragement of the private circulation, discouraging the savings etc., is not clearly known. This is the present situation and scenario.

Principles of Taxation

Tax is the important source of the Pubic Finance. Tax can not be collected from the people, units, organisations etc just like that i.e with out any policy and strategy. Also it should not be. The responsible authority (may be single person or group of persons) first understand the fundamental truths of the tax, fundamental purpose of the tax and the meaning of the tax. This is called the Principles of tax. A tax policy made without the knowledge of the principles of tax will create a lot of confusions, imbalances, and quantitative and qualitative ups and downs in the status of individuals. In fact these are the serious issues and causes for the adverse development economically and socially. So a good tax structure and policy should have the following Principles.

1. Tax Structure/Policy should increases the Resources for the economic development.
2. Tax Structure/Policy should promote the savings and investment.
3. Tax Structure/Policy should reduce the inequalities.
4. Tax Structure/Policy should compel the government to reduce the heavy present government expenditure.
5. Tax Structure/Policy should directly or indirectly increase the efficiency of the people.
6. Tax Structure/Policy must not be a complex one. It must be simple to calculate and easy to understand.
7. Tax Structure/Policy should not be always unfaithful
8. Tax Structure/Policy should be impartial.

Some of the above principles are discussed below. This is also given in illustrative form.

Principles of Increasing Resources

Financial resources are very important for all the Economic activities of the country. No finance means no development. To develop the country economically and to maintain the economic stability, any country needs the revenue i.e Public Revenue. So the tax structure/policy is to be constructed in such a way that the government must get more revenue or income either directly or indirectly to increase the resource with out burdening the people. The responsible people must see the ways and means to collect tax every year. This will be like to pluck the rose from the plants in such a way the garden should be with the full of roses and each plant also should have roses. It is not like that plucking all roses from one or two plants by leaving the other plants untouched. So the Tax Structure/Policy must be as per the above truth.

Principles of Promoting Savings and Investments

"Savings" is one of the factors determining the economic growth. More savings mean more growth. No savings means no growth. Savings are an important element of social system. Savings are the roots of the investment trees. The investments are the trees that will provide all sorts of benefits to the society including the maintenance of environment and rain stability. Once the savings are stopped and are not encouraged, the corresponding effects will be seen in the output of investment tree. Even a layman can easily understand the above effect when there is no investment. Hence, Tax Structure/Policy must always aim the growth of investment. For that purpose, Tax Structure/Policy must encourage the savings.

Principle of Equality

This is very important principle yet to be taken into consideration in the Tax Structure/Policy. Knowingly or unknowingly, I don't know, why the principle of equality is, totally, being omitted in the present setup of the tax organisation. May be, specified groups are benefitted, the reason for such omission of principle. We have been seeing that among the salaried group of taxpayers, the families with Single Earner (SE) will have a lot of problems than that of the families with Double Earners (DE). The DE group will always enjoys the benefits of social up-ness due to more income. They will be living with Car, TV, VCR, sophisticated furniture, costly dresses, and cosmopolitan life by gaining the society's attractions with a very big circle. Whereas the families with the SE though they are trying with a lot of hardship, they can not due to their limited inflow of cash into the family. The DE group has been enjoying the multiple benefits of the Standard Deduction, additional tax rebate benefit of Rs. 5000 to the wife, the family gets total deduction of Rs. 50,000 and total tax rebate of Rs. 30,000 with the savings facilities of Rs. 200000 etc., as far as the tax payment is concerned.

Another touching important point is that the impacts of such groups will be reflected upon the children of the groups. Though the expenditure per family of these two groups are more or less same, it is quiet natural, the SE group will face the problem in satisfying their children even to provide the basic needs. But the DE group will go by four wheelers due to their more savings and more inflow of cash inside the family. In short, they acquire a special status in the society whereas, as is already told, the SE group has to be always like oil on a water in the society. Moreover, the society itself will corner such SE in the long run. The people under the DE group will not like this article because they feel this article contain something against that group. But what is written is the fact and that too real fact practically going in the present world/society. So the Tax structure/Policy should have the Principle of Equity with a view to avoid inequalities in the society. The learned readers are requested not to misinterpret that the author is against the DE group. To give a suggestion for the tax reform, this is quoted as an example.

Principles of Taxation and Tax Reform

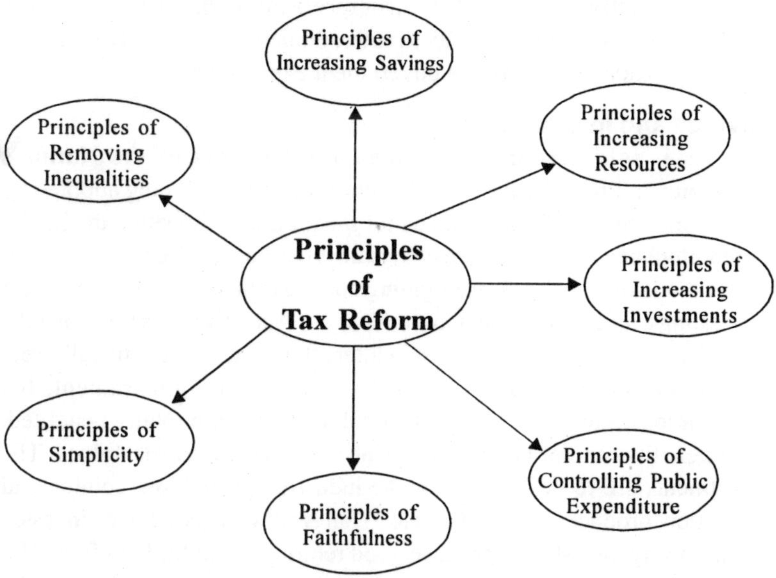

Fig. 02

Principles of Controlled Expenses

To be very frank, the day to day business of the government is being transacted out of the public revenue/finance for which the major portion (almost full) comes from the tax. Tax in a sensible sense, is a portion of hard earned money of the people. But in a orthodox sense, it is the major portion of the sacrifice of the persons. But, now we see what is actually going in the countries of the world. The major portion of the Public Finance is being and is to be spent on the securities for the individual leader/politicians. Unproductive wages are being paid when some meaningless and baseless problems created by the politicians by other leaders. The unplanned way of administration and management of the less efficient officers compels the government to pay for the unproductive payments. Delay on the part of the govt.,. employees particularly at the higher level in taking decision due to their inability and less knowledge, the government has to spend more money for the unproductive wages; wrong perception of the "Concept of Government Employment" and absence of the "Systematic Management" bring unnecessary conflicts and thereby the payments made to the employees automatically become the unproductive. So the Tax structure/Policy should control the government expenditure. The Tax structure/Policy must suggest the various ways and means to control the government expenditure

Savings and Investments

As is told earlier, the savings are the roots of the Nation's development. Presently the "savings and tax system" is being adopted by the government. Tax is being taken for the purpose of meeting the public expenditure and the savings are being taken for the purpose of investment. Again the investment has been giving some earnings to the government by creating a lot employment opportunities etc. Actually this is the principle. Even if this is not followed, at least in future this principle is to be followed. The person or persons who save for savings, the government, the organisations, the public sector undertakings, etc., are totally benefited. Such benefits can not be measured since they have intrinsic values. The investments are to be utilised for the industrial promotion, commercial promotion, productive promotion etc., That is, all savings are to be invested in such a way they should produce good return with multiplier effect. If it is not invested in a prudent way, then there is no use of having the investment and all such savings will go waste. If the savings are removed from the Tax structure/Policy, what will happen? The employees will not go for savings with the government schemes since the rate of interest is low. Naturally, it will tempt them to go for the private investment like money lending business, kenthu interest business, finance business, cheetu business, and what not. The concentration of the people will be more in their money circulation than that of their job concentration. Now the present situation is very worst because the concentration of the employees in jobs has been gradually coming down and that's why the government is thinking seriously to go for privatisation. Then the situation may arise that the government may go to private individuals for financial assistance in the form of loan etc. which will not be a good symptom for a developing country.

Standard Deduction

Actually the Standard Deduction means the deduction allowed by the Income Tax Act to the individual assess to meet their incidental expenses. This has a strong association with the employment particularly those which do not provide amenities like motor car, provisions of the free cook, watchman, gardener etc. The dangerous, in removing and standard deduction and savings, and keeping the maximum tax-free limit before such standard deduction and savings, is to be foreseen. If the standard deduction is removed and savings are discouraged, naturally, the persons will have more money (unsaved i.e money kept for the savings). If the employee go for three months leave with loss of pay, there are chances, his income will come down to a considerable level. He can escape from the tax liability. Again the particular office will have problems due to fewer staff. To complete the work, problems of overtime, etc will automatically increase the pressure on the head of the office. Under any circumstances, the Standard Deduction may not be removed at the interest of the taxpayers and the government.

Need for the Tax Reform

There is an absolute need for the tax reform at this hour and it should continue every year without disturbing the previous announcements. For example, last year only, the government announced the provisions related to the accrued interest on the House Building Advance/Loan. But now the thinking of disclaiming the same create something like unfaithfulness in the brain of the taxpayers. Many times this has happened in case of Jeevan Dhara, NSS etc. This type of practice is to be totally avoided. It is not criticized but before taking a decision, the matters are to be analysed and thought of many times. One man should not be allowed to take a decision. In the same manner, a specified group of vested interest people alone should not be asked to give opinion. It is clearly mentioned in the principles of taxation that the Tax Structure/Policy should aim at the increase of resources, reduction of the inequalities, increase the savings and investments and to control the government expenditure. All these principles must be present in the Tax Policy. But the present Tax Structure is not of full fledged. It lacks some of the important principles. So there is an absolute need for the Tax Reform.

Concept of Family Assessment

Next to the Principles of taxation, in the process of the tax reform, introduction of new concepts in the tax structure and policy is very much essential. One has to take the current economic situation of our country, social imbalances, social inequalities and allied problems, possible ways of multiplying the income and allied effectivity, and unemployment problems and allied affectivity. Tax reform can not satisfy all people always. There must be definitely some criticisms to this new concept. More over this concept should not be confused with the concept of Hindu Undivided

Family (HUF) and Joint Hindu Family (JHF). The nature and feature of HUF & JHF are entirely different from the newly proposed Concept of Family Assessment. So as a new concept, the Family Assessment is to be introduced. Instead of calculating inflow of money (income) in the hands of individuals the inflow of money in to the family is to be taken for the purpose of tax computation. For example, if in a family X, "A" is the husband gets his income Rs. 2,00,000,and "B" the wife Rs. 2,00,000. In another family Y, the husband "C" gets his income Rs. 2,00,000 and the wife does not go for job. As per the principles of Taxation as is discussed before, Family X is called as DE Group and the Family Y is called as SE Group. The total inflow of the cash/money into the family X is Rs. 4,00,000 whereas into the family Y it is only Rs. 2,00,000. Now Mr. A, Mrs. B and Mr. C are assessed for tax individually on their income. As such these three assesses have to pay the tax. Mr. A will have to pay a net tax of Rs. 10,000 (i.e. 5.8% of his income after SD) his wife B will have to pay a net tax of Rs. 5,000 (i.e.2.9% of her income after SD) and the Mr. C will have to pay Rs. 14,500 (i.e. 8.5%of his income after SD) and these are 5.0%; 2.5%; and 7.25% respectively on Gross Salary. Here the assumption made is that the expenditure for these two families are the same and the number of members in these two families are also the same. Mr. A and his wife Mrs. B save Rs. 2,00,000 i.e each Rs. 1,00,000 (Rs. 70,000 + 30,000) due to the fact that the inflow of cash into their family is more whereas the Mr. C could not save that much due to the fact that the inflow of cash into his family is less however with great difficulties he is able to save atleast Rs. 70,000. It is quiet natural that family X will always be with more amount of money circulation than that of family Y both in the future as well as at present. The total tax to the government is Rs.29,500 if the tax is assessed individually. There are a lot of social imbalances. The family X gets the following benefits:

1. Double Standard Deduction of Rs 60,000 (Rs.30,000 + 30,000)
2. Double Maximum Tax Free Limit i.e Rs. 1,00,000 (Rs. 50,000 + .50,000)
3. Special Deduction for Female Assessee Rs. 5,000 directly from the Tax
4. Benefits of Future Investment Return – Double ROI-Return On Investment.
5. Double Investment Return facilitate the family X to go for further money circulations, and multiple investment schemes.

Whereas the family Y gets nothing. The benefits enjoyed by the DE

Families and the calculations of the tax liabilities are given in the Illustrative Tables "IT-A" and "IT-B" Suppose if the new concept of family assessment is introduced, as per the calculation mentioned in the suggestion (please see the suggestion), the family X has to make the payment of tax on the family income of Rs. 4,00,000. They will have Rs. 50,000 (justified) as the standard deduction and thereby their income tax liability will come Rs.64,000. This is only 18.3% of their total income after SD and the same is only 16.0% of family income before the SD. . Now the introduction of the Concept of Family Assessment, the government will get tax revenue of Rs. 78,500. The family Y of SE Group with the income of Rs. 2,00,000, SD benefit of Rs. 30,000 savings limitation of Rs. 70,000 pays tax to the government Rs. 14,500 i.e. at the rate of 8.5%of his income after SD. Whereas the Family X of DE Group with the income of Rs. 4,00,000, SD benefit of Rs. 50,000, savings limitation of Rs. 1, 00,000 pays tax to the government Rs. 64,000 i.e. 18.3% of the family income after SD and the same is only 16.0% of family income before the SD. Here one can understand the justification of introducing the new concept of Family Assessment is that the family "Y" with Single Earner(SE) pays 8.5% of family income after SD and a family "X" with Double Earners(DE) pays 18.3% (i.e. progressive) of family income after SD. The government gets more benefit of getting increased revenue. Social imbalances will go down to some extent, unemployment problem will be solved to some extent etc. This is shown in the table form.

Illustrative Table "IT – A"

Sl. No.	*Particulars*	*Family "X" Husband (Rs.)*	*Family "X" Wife (Rs.)*	*Family "Y" Husband (Rs.)*
1	Gross Salary	2,00,000	2,00,000	2,00,000
2	Standard Deduction	30,000	30,000	30,000
3	Taxable Salary	1,70,000	1,70,000	1,70,000
4	Tax at Present Rate	25,000	25,000	25,000
5	Rebate at Present Rat	15,000	15,000	10,500
6	Gross Tax Payable	10,000	10,000	14,500
7	Special Tax Relief on Sex	Nil	5,000	Nil
8	Net Tax Payable	10,000	5,000	14,500
9	%of Net Tax before SD	5.0%	2.5%	7.25%
10	% of Net Tax after SI	5.8%	2.9%	8.5%

Illustrative Table "IT-B"
Benefits Enjoyed by the Families of Double Earnings (DE) and Single Earnings(SE)

Sl. No.	*Particulars & Benefits*	*Family "X" Double Earnings (Rs.)*	*Family "Y" Single Earnings(Rs.)*
01	Total Income of the Family	4,00,000	4,00,000
02	Benefits Enjoyed		
(a)	Standard Deduction	60,000	30,000
(b)	Maximum Tax Free Limit	1,00,000	50,000
(c)	Rebate	30,000	10,500
(c)	Special Rebate on Tax	5,000	Nil
(d)	Savings/Investments	2,00,000	70,000
(e)	Interest on Savings @ 9%	Per Year 18,000	Per Year 6,300
(f)	Total Benefit on Spot	3,95,000	1,60,500
	% of Benefits on Total Income	98.75%	40.12%
	Every Year Future Benefits	Rs. 18,000	Rs. 6,300
(f)	Tax Payable	15,000	14,500
(g)	% Tax on total inflow of cash into the family	3.75%	7.25%

Table 1
Comparative Assessment of DE Group & SE Group in two families

Sl. No.	*Particulars*	*Family X DE Group*	*Family Y SE Group*	*Revenue to Govt. (Rs.)*
1	Number of Members Husband, Wife and Three Children	05	05	---
2	Number of Earning Members	02 Husband & Wife	01 Husband	----
3	Income Per Head @ Rs. 200000	4,00,000	2,00,000	----
4	Standard Deduction @ Rs. 30,000 (At Present Structure - APS)	60,000	30,000	----
5	Savings for the Tax Rebate-APS	2,00,000	70,000	----
6	Tax Rebate General- APS	30,000	10,500	----
7	Tax Rebate for Female- APS	5,000	----	----
8	Total Tax Rebate- APS	35,000	10,500	-----

Sl. No.	Particulars	Family X DE Group	Family Y SE Group	Revenue to Govt. (Rs.)
9	Net Tax (APS)	15,000 10,000+ 5,000	14,500	29,500

Source: Calculated and Computed

Table 2
Assessment of DE Group Family "N" and SE Group Family "R" Whose inflow of the Cash is Rs. 4,00,000 As per the Present way of Assessment

Sl. No.	Particulars	Family N DE Group	Family R SE Group	Revenue to Govt. (Rs.)
1	Number of Members Husband, Wife and Three Children	05	05	---
2	Number of Earning Members	02 Husband & Wife	01 Husband	----
3	Income Per Head @ Rs. 200000 for Family N and Rs. 400000 for Family R	4,00,000	4,00,000	----
4	Standard Deduction @ Rs.30,000 (At Present Structure - APS)	60,000	30,000	----
5	Savings for the Tax Rebate- APS	2,00,000	1,00,000	----
6	Tax Rebate General- APS	30,000	15,000	----
7	Tax Rebate for Female- APS	5,000	----	----
8	Total Tax Rebate- APS	35,000	15,000	---
9	Net Tax (APS)	15,000 10,000+ 5000	70,000	85,000
10	% of Net Tax on Income after S.D	4.4%	18.9%	
11	% of Net Tax on Income before S.D	3.75%	17.5%	

Source: Calculated and Computed

Table 3
Comparative Assessment of Income on the basis of the Suggested Concept of Family Assessment

S.No	Particulars	Family N DE Group	Family R SE Group	Revenue to Govt. (Rs.)
1	Number of Members Husband, Wife and Three Children	05	05	---

S.No	Particulars	Family N DE Group	Family R SE Group	Revenue to Govt. (Rs.)
2	Number of Earning Members	02 Husband & Wife	01 Husband	----
3	Income Per Head @ Rs. 200000	4,00,000	4,00,000	----
4	Standard Deduction @ Rs.30,000 rate (At Present Structure – APS)	50,000	30,000	----
5	Savings for the Tax Rebate- APS	1,00,000	1,00,000	----
6	Tax Rebate General- APS	15,000	15,000	----
7	Tax Rebate for Female- APS	----	----	----
8	Total Tax Rebate- APS	15,000	15,000	-----
9	Net Tax (APS)	64,000	70,000	1,34,000
10	% of Net Tax on Income after S.D	18.3%	18.9%	
11	% of Net Tax on Income before S.D	21.0%	17.5%	

Source: Calculated and Computed.

Analysation of the present tax structure

With the help of the above table the present tax structure is analysed here. Table 01 gives the comparative assessment of Individuals in the Family X and in the Family Y on the basis of individual assessment. Family X and Family Y, both are equal in family size, in the expenditure range and in social obligations. In family Y only the husband goes for Job i.e. only the husband is able to go for job due to the unemployment problems whereas in family X both husband and wife go for job. Here the assumption is that all Mr. A, Mrs.B of family X and Mr. C of the family Y get the same amount of salary/income say Rs. 2,00,000 p.a. If they are assessed individually:

Mr. A has to pay a tax of	Rs. 10,000	
Mrs. B has to pay a tax of	Rs. 5,000	Rs. 15,000
Mr. C has to pay tax of		Rs. 14,500
The Tax revenue to the Government		Rs. 29,500

It is already mentioned the benefits enjoyed by the family X. But the contradiction here is that the provisions of the Income Tax seem to be partial incase of the family with one person going for job. Because a family (DE Group) which is getting Rs. 4,00,000 as its income pays only Rs. 15,000 (Just 3.75%)as tax where as a family (SE Group) which is getting Rs. 2,00,000 as its income pays Rs.14,500 (7.25%). So the author feels that there is no Justice.

Now the Table 02 gives the comparative assessment of the Family X consisting of husband Mr. A and wife Mrs. B and another family Z consisting of husband Mr. D and wife Mrs. E. Here is also in family Z only one person i.e. husband Mr. D goes for but he earns Rs. 4,00,000 p.a. Family wise, these two families get the same amount of inflow of cash i.e the same income. But, if they are assessed for tax as per the present structure individually,

Mr. A has to pay a tax of	Rs. 10,000	
Mrs. B has to pay a tax of	Rs. 5,000	Rs. 15,000
Mr. D has to pay tax of		Rs. 70,000
The Tax revenue to the Government		Rs. 85,000

It is already mentioned the benefits enjoyed by the family "X". But the contradiction here is that the provisions of the Income Tax seem to be partial at high level incase of the family "Z" also with one person going for job. Because a family "X" (DE Group) which is getting Rs. 4,00,000 as its income pays only Rs. 15,000 (Just3.75%)as tax where as a family "Z" (SE Group) which is also getting Rs. 4,00,000 as its income pays Rs.70,000 (17.5%). So the author feels that there is no Justice in this case also.

One has to seriously think that one man earns Rs. 4,00,000 and he helps rather is asked to help the government resource by contributing Rs. 70,000 whereas two persons earn the same amount but they are asked to pay only Rs. 15,000. Such a long and vast injustice require justice. Even by combining the table 01, the family X with DE Group by enjoying a lot of qualitative and quantitative benefits from the government and by creating heavy social imbalance pays very less tax. Hence the author proposes the new concept to be introduced into the Tax Policy and the Tax Structure in the name of the Tax Reform. The author is ready to clarify the doubts of anybody as far as the new concept of Family assessment is concerned. Hence by comparing the family X (DE Group) and family Z (SE Group) an assessment has been made at the present rates but on the basis of the newly proposed Concept of Family Assessment and presented in Table 03. Here the family X is given an additional benefit of Standard Deduction i.e. Rs. 50,000. Total cash inflow into the families in the name of income is taken for the calculation. As such:

Family X will have to pay a tax of	Rs. 64,000
Family Z will have to pay a tax of	Rs. 70,000
The government will get revenue	Rs.134,000

Justification

1. The Concept of Family Assessment is a newly proposed suggestive Assessment.
2. Families with SE Group are not all affected.
3. Families with DE Group contribute more to the Public Revenue on the basis of More Income More Tax and vice versa.
4. It is a type of progressive tax suggestion and progressive suggestion.
5. There may be strong criticism from the side of the DE group. But if they think seriously about the welfare of our Country in all dimensions and go through this article, there will not be any problem to implement the newly proposed concept.
6. The Social Imbalances will be reduced and inequalities will be removed.
7. There are chances for the increasing employment opportunities in long run.
8. Standard Deduction for the Family Assessment (DE Group) is fixed at Rs. 50,000.
9. Strong Rules are to be made and they are to be managed very carefully and without partiality. As far as the disclosure of income is concerned all the employees should necessarily declare the required information. That is possible through the strict disciplinary actions and crystal clear manual rules.

Concept of Tax Saving Fund

As is told in the Principles of Taxation, savings are the pillars of the Nation's Development. Now to save tax i.e. to get tax rebate the assessees have to save in the LIC, NSC, PPF, GPF, ULIP, Mutual Funds, ICICI Bonds, Home Loan Account under the National Housing Scheme etc. Instead of asking the people to go for different savings schemes, a common fund may be set up with the rules and regulations. So the government may go for the common fund in the name of Tax Saving Fund (TSF) with the following rules and regulations.

1. Any amount deposited in the TSF qualifies for the Tax Rebate
2. The Deposit in the TSF will earn an interest @ 9% p.a. compounded half yearly and the government should not further reduce the rate of Interest atleast for TSF.
3. The interest accrued in TSF is totally exempt from tax.
4. The Assessee can withdraw any amount only after the expiry of the 10th year from the date of the initial deposit.
5. If the assessee wish to avail a loan against the TSF/out of TSF,

he will be given a loan upto 75% of the deposit for the interest @ 11% p.a. compounded yearly which will be automatically deducted from his salary with out his consent.

6. The government can ask any of its department or it can ask any banker to manage this fund. Necessary instructions are to be given to the DDOs regarding this matter otherwise, they will ride the horse.
7. The present limit of the qualifying amount of Rs. 70, 000 plus Rs. 30,000 with the 15% tax rebate may be increased to Rs.1,00,000 in TSF with the 20% tax rebate with NO surcharge.

Identifying and Enlisting the New Assesses

Next aspect of the management of the tax reform is to identify and enlist the new assessees who earn money in uncountable level. They are to be brought in the tax assesses list. The authorities must take all possible steps to identify such type of hidden money minters. For example, Kenthu interest business people are very well visible in the society but they are not taken for the assessment. Individuals engaging private tuitions, coaching Centres etc., are not fully brought into the assessment list but they are to be brought under the accounts and they are to be ordered to pay the tax. This is because, for example, an individual private tutor charges heavily from the students. Since the DE group does not mind to pay so much of the amount and the SE Group is also compelled to pay the same money. Since the tuition has become a fashion now a days, the private tuition Centres are minting money like anything. The prevailing rates are given below:

1.	For Language	from Class KG to Class IV	Rs. 150.00 PH., PM., Psub.,
2.	For Main Subject	from Class KG to Class IV	Rs. 200.00 PH., PM., Psub.,
3.	For Language	from Class V to Class VII	Rs. 200.00 PH., PM., Psub.,
4.	For Main Subject	from Class V to Class VII	Rs. 250.00 PH., PM., Psub.,
5.	For Language	from Class VIII to Class X	Rs 250.00 PH., PM., Psub.,
6.	For Main Subject	from Class VIII to Class X	Rs. 300.00 PH., PM., Psub.,
7.	For all Arts subjects	for Class XI & XII	Rs. 300.00 PH., PM., Psub.,
8.	For Mathematics	for Class XI & XII	Rs. 400.00 PH., PM., Psub.,
9.	For all Sci.Subjects	for Class XI & XII	Rs. 500.00 PH., PM., Psub.,

PH – Per Head, PM-Per Month and Psub- Per Subject.

Per month means full month but the classes will be conducted by the tuition masters only in alternative days. It is calculated that these masters are engaging classes in terms of batches. Normally they engage 3 batches morning hours and 3 batches evening hours except Sundays. In total they call for 6 batches per day for 6 days i.e 6x6 = 36 batches per week i.e 36 x 4 = 144 batches per month. Each batch consists of on an average 20 students claiming 144x20 = 2880 students per month. The charge for the calculation purpose is taken Rs. 300PM PH, Psub. This comes around Rs. 8,64,000 PM. Their earning per year will be around 1 Crore. This is only a layman calculation with the help of information available. The income tax department must send their inspectors to collect information. They are to be brought under the regulation.

Suggestions

Tax is necessary to meet all the government expenditure for the betterment of the public at large. The principles of the taxation have been discussed in the previous paras. Taxation must aim at the increasing the public revenue without making the tax payers tired. The majority of the people should unanimously accept it though not by all. The tax reform is to be made in such way that it should automatically reduce the inequality among the people of same categories. The Following suggestions are offered to manage the Tax Structure which is Tax Reform is the need of the hour to our country. Since this piece of work is related to only the individual taxpayers the suggestions are also restricted to only those areas which will surround the salaried group of the people and individual taxpayers.

1. Tax Reform must be thought of completely on the basis of the Principles of Taxation given in this piece of work. It is suggested that one should not think only in one way without giving opportunities to others to hear and give their suggestions. Tax Reform is having a long way to decide by taking all the relevant points and convenience of the person paying the tax.
2. Tax reforms must always be forward oriented. Giving one concession in one year and removing the concession in the next year by introducing some unrelated issues in the year concerned are not considered as tax reforms. Such practices must be totally avoided since the people will loose their confidence not only on the government but also on the Income Tax.
3. Now in the name of Tax Reform, many talks are going like the standard deduction is to be removed, discourage of savings, removal of the House Building Advance/Loan's interest accumulation in the assessment of income etc. It is suggested as not to disturb the Standard Deduction, not to discourage the savings that are the roots of the Investments and capital mobilization. In fact the standard deduction is the privileged deduction available for the salaried group

to meet their incidental expenses. Hence, it should not be set aside under any circumstances. Savings are like the iron rods inside the investment-concreted Nation Building. If the savings are discouraged, the building will collapse soon. So it is highly warned that our interest payment will go up. One should seriously think about the different ways by which the collected savings may be invested to earn further income.

4. No doubt, the government has removed the surcharge for the assessment year 2004-05 but it is suggested that the Surcharges are to be totally removed. This is because, the persons are already overloaded with the payment of income tax and for every purchase, they are compelled and forced to make the indirect taxes. The business people, by transferring the tax burden upon the customers (individuals) in the name of indirect taxes, do escape from their responsibilities. Their margin is always assured to them and ultimate sufferers are our poor individual taxpayers. It is suggested to remove the surcharge.

5. At present the tax is being collected only from the government employees and some employees of the private sector. Number of persons to be included in the list of assessees is knowingly or unknowingly being omitted. Many people whose income is more than the maximum tax free limit do escape from the responsibility of paying income tax since there is no mechanism to find out their income. For example, the coaching centres, individuals engaging in the private tuitions, money lenders, Kenthu interest money lenders, commission agents, private traders etc. These are only examples. Like wise, there are plenty of people, associations, groups, and uncovered contractors to be included in the list. Actually it is the duty of the Inspectors of Income Tax to go to different places to collect the information about the people who are coming under the tax paying brackets.

6. Now the MLAs and MPs are given monthly salary like other government employees. Hence, the concessions, special rebates, exemptions, limits etc., are to be stopped and they should also be assessed like other assesses with the compulsion to disclose all the properties.

7. Now the income tax is calculated on the basis of the individual income particularly in the salaried group, individuals are very much specific. In a house, both the husband and wife are going for job means,

husband is taxed for his own income and like that the wife's. This is the major area requires reformation. Instead of calculating the income tax on the income of a person(individual), income tax is to be calculated on the income of the family (Husband and Wife). That is, instead of calculating the inflow of the cash/income to an individual's pocket as taxable income for the purpose of computing the tax, it is highly suggested that the inflow of the cash/income into the family is to be calculated as taxable income for the purpose of computation of income tax.

8. It is expected that there will be a lot of opposition from the side of the family wherein both the husband and wife are going for job. I knew that definitely there will be resistance for this suggestion. Hence, it is suggested that when the income of the husband and the income of the wife is added for the determination of the taxable income, a combined standard deduction may be given. For example, now the standard deduction per individual is 40% or 30,000 whichever is less is given. But for the family assessment, the standard deduction may be 40% or 50,000 whichever is less may be given and it is suggested so. As far as the tax rate is concerned, there should not be any change for the family assessment. Maximum Tax Free Limit, Tax Rebates, Tax Rates applicable for the individuals (i.e Single Earner Group) are to be made applicable to the family assessment also (i.e Double Earners Group). The officers or the employees have to sincerely declare the fact about the spouse. Suppressing the facts has to attract severe punishment. One should seriously think about this suggestion at the interest of the Nation. To some extent, this will help the government to solve the unemployment problem also.

9. There should not be any dual treatment between assessees on the basis of sex. In front of tax calculation everybody should be treated at par and equally. So a special deduction or the rebate for the female sex may be removed at the interest of the nation.

10. By taking all the points in to consideration, it is suggested that maximum tax free limit may be raised from Rs. 50,000 to 80,000. The monetary limit of Standard Deduction may be increased from Rs.30,000 or 40 % to 40,000 or 40% whichever is less for the individuals i.e SE Group and Rs. 50,000 or 40% whichever is less for the family assessment i.e DE Group. That is, the Standard Deduction may be 40% of the Gross Salary or Rs. 40,000 whichever is less and for the proposed family assessment for the DE group the Standard Deduction may be 40% of the total Gross Salary of Family (i.e Income

of the Husband and the income of the Wife are to be totaled) or 50,000 whichever is less.

11. It is suggested that the government may go for a concept of Tax Saving Fund (TSF) with the rules and regulations for the withdrawals only after 10 years may be setup. The present limit of the qualifying amount of Rs. 70, 000 plus Rs. 30,000 with the 15% tax rebate & 5% surcharge may be increased to Rs.1,00,000 in TSF with the 20% tax rebate with NO surcharge.

12. The Higher Income Group i.e individuals or families may be excluded from such concessions and tax rebates. That is, an individual or a family whose annual income is more than Rs. 4,50,000 before the Standard Deduction but after the deduction of income exempt under section 10 may be given only standard deduction but not any tax rebate, and an individual or a family whose annual income is more than Rs. 5,00,000 before the Standard Deduction but after the deduction of income exempt under section 10 may not be given any deduction and tax rebates and they should pay tax on their Salary income.

13. The following Tax rates are suggested:

	Income from (Rs.)		*Income to (Rs.)*	*Rate in %1.*
1.	Rs.	01	80,000	Nil
2.	Rs.	80,001	Rs. 1,00,000	10%
3.	Rs.	1,00,001	Rs. 2,50,000	20%
4.	Rs.	2,50,001	and above	30%
5.	Surcharge: -		NIL	

Here the income means, the Income from Salary after the Standard Deduction, after the set-off of the accrued interest on the House Building Advance as per the existing rule and after the deduction under chapter VI (as usual what is going at present)

14. The balance of tax to be collected from the individuals like actors, artists, politicians, etc., are to be collected as early as possible. Steps are to be taken to collect such balances. The politician who has the balance of tax to the government is not to be allowed to context in any election. If any law permits such politicians to context, the law is to be amended immediately. Even if they are in any responsible post, the balance of tax is to be collected.

Conclusion

The above suggestions, principles and concepts are to be placed before the balanced learned persons, impartial experts, experienced economists, Nation Loving Patriotic to elicit their valuable analysation and approval in the name of the seminar and discussions. The above writings are only my views for the further analysation. Once if the tax policy/structure is constructed as per the Principles of Taxation mentioned above, the Concepts of Family Assessment and the of Tax Saving Fund are introduced and in the light of the above suggestions in the name of Tax Reform and if it is managed properly, I am sure that the inequalities among the salaried group will be removed to some extent, unemployment problems will be solved to some extent, Savings and Investments will be increased considerably and the public finance will go up certainly which will raise the fiscal resources. Such Management of Tax Reform will convert our Indian Economy from the word "Developing" into the word "Developed".

36

Need for the Concept of Family Assessment in Tax Reform

Introduction

Every country gets its revenue in two ways namely Tax Revenue and Non- Tax Revenue. Tax revenue includes direct taxes (Income Tax, Wealth Tax, Gift Tax, Entertainment tax, etc.) and indirect tax (sales tax, customs duties, excise duties etc.) Non tax revenues includes the revenues from the public undertakings. Among these two sources, the Tax revenue constitutes the major portion. The tax policy should have social and economic objectives, which will differ, from one country to other country. The tax system and structure should not be a mere leap in the dark. So, depending upon the economic situation prevailing in the country, the tax system, structure and policy are to be constructed. This process is called Tax reform. In the process of the Tax Reform new concepts are to be brought in by giving more importance to the social and economic objectives. Discussions and measures given in this paper are only suggestions. Accepting or rejecting is absolutely in the hands of the learned people and the government.

Changes Brought by the Finance Bill 2003

The finance minister Jaswant Singh in the parliament presented the Union Budget 2003-04 on 28th Feb., 2003. The important changes brought in are that the standard deduction limit has been raised from Rs. 25,000 to 40% or Rs. 30,000, whichever is less for those earning below Rs. 5 lakh per annum. But if the annual salary is over Rs. 5 lakh, then your standard deduction limit has been reduced to Rs. 20,000. The 5% surcharge levied in last budget has been removed for individuals. The total deduction of

Rs. 9,000 earlier available under section 80L with regard to income from dividend and interest has been upped to Rs. 12,000. Interest rate on investment in PPF and small savings has been further reduced by 1% from March 2003. Indian citizens have to compulsorily furnish PAN numbers for foreign travel. Procedures and methods for search and seizure operations during income tax survey have been simplified and individual taxpayers have to fill single-page income-tax return form for filing IT returns.

Need for the Tax Reform

There is an absolute need for the tax reform at this hour and it should continue every year without disturbing the previous announcement. The Tax Structure/Policy should aim at the increase of resources, reduction of the inequalities, increase the savings and investments and to control the government expenditure. All these principles must be present in the Tax Policy. But the present Tax Structure is not of full fledged. It lacks some of the important principles. So there is an absolute need for the Tax Reform.

Concept of Family Assessment

In the process of the tax reform, introduction of new concepts in the tax structure and policy is very much essential. One has to take the current economic situation of our country, social imbalances, social inequalities and allied problems, possible ways of multiplying the income and allied effectivity, and unemployment problems and allied affectivity. Tax reform can not satisfy all people always. There must be definitely some criticisms to this new concept. More over this concept should not be confused with the concept of Hindu Undivided Family (HUF) and Joint Hindu Family (JHF). The nature and feature of HUF & JHF are entirely different from the newly proposed Concept of Family Assessment. So as a new concept, the Family Assessment is necessarily to be introduced in the present tax structure.

Explanation

The Concept of Family Assessment is a new concept in which instead of calculating inflow of money (income) in the hands of individuals the inflow of money in to the family is to be taken for the purpose of tax computation. For example, if in a family X, "A" is the husband gets his income Rs. 2,00,000,and "B" the wife Rs. 2,00,000. In another family Y, the husband "C" gets his income Rs. 2,00,000 and the wife does not go for job. The Family X is called as Double Earning Group i.e DE Group and the Family Y is called as Single Earning Group i.e SE Group. The total inflow of the cash/money into the family X is Rs. 4,00,000 whereas into the family Y it is only Rs. 2,00,000. Now Mr. A, Mrs. B and Mr. C are assessed for tax individually on their income. As such these three assess have to pay the tax. Mr. A will have to pay a net tax of Rs. 10,000 (i.e. 5.8% of his income after SD) his wife B will have to pay a net tax of Rs. 5,000 (i.e.2.9% of her income after SD) and the Mr. C will have to pay Rs. 14,500 (i.e. 8.5%of his income after SD) and these are 5.0%; 2.5%; and 7.25% respectively on Gross Salary. This is given in Table 01. Here the assumption made is that the expenditure for these two families are the same and the number of members in these two families are also the same. Mr. A and his wife Mrs. B save Rs. 2,00,000 i.e each Rs. 1,00,000 (Rs. 70,000 + 30,000) due to the fact that the inflow of cash into their family is more whereas the Mr. C could not save that much due to the fact that the inflow of cash into his family is less however with great difficulties he is able to save atleast Rs. 70,000. It is quiet natural that family X will always be with more amount of money circulation than that of family Y both in the future as well as at present. The total tax to the government is Rs.29,500 if the tax is assessed individually. There are a lot of social imbalances. The family X gets the following benefits:

1. Double Standard Deduction of Rs 60,000 (Rs.30,000 + 30,000)
2. Double Maximum Tax Free Limit. i.e., Rs. 1,00,000 (Rs. 50,000 + 50,000)
3. Special Deduction for Female Assessee Rs. 5,000 directly from the Tax
4. Benefits of Future Investment Return – Double ROI-Return On Investment.
5. Double Investment Return facilitate the family X to go for further money circulations, and multiple investment schemes.

Whereas the family Y gets nothing. The benefits enjoyed by the DE Families and are given in the Tables 2 Suppose if the new concept of family assessment is introduced, as per the calculation mentioned in the suggestion (please see the suggestion), the family X has to make the payment of tax on the family income of Rs. 4,00,000. They will have Rs. 50,000 (justified) as the standard deduction and thereby their income tax liability will come Rs. 64,000. This is only 18.3% of their total income after SD and the same is only 16.0% of family income before the SD.

Now the introduction of the Concept of Family Assessment, the government will get tax revenue of Rs. 78,500. The family Y of SE Group with the income of Rs. 2,00,000, SD benefit of Rs. 30,000 savings limitation of Rs. 70,000 pays tax to the government Rs. 14,500 i.e. at the rate of 8.5% of his income after SD. Whereas the Family X of DE Group with the income of Rs. 4,00,000, SD benefit of Rs. 50,000, savings limitation of Rs. 1, 00,000 pays tax to the government Rs. 64,000, i.e., 18.3% of the family income after

SD and the same is only 16.0% of family income before the SD. Here one can understand the justification of introducing the New Concept of Family Assessment is that the family "Y" with Single Earner(SE) pays 8.5% of family income after SD and a family "X" with Double Earners(DE) pays 18.3% (i.e. progressive) of family income after SD. The government gets more benefit of getting increased revenue. Social imbalances will go down to some extent, unemployment problem will be solved to some extent etc. This is shown in the table form.

Table 1
Individual Assessments

Sl. No.	*Particulars*	*Family "X" Husband (Rs.)*	*Family "X" Wife (Rs.)*	*Family "Y" Husband (Rs.)*
1	Gross Salary	2,00,000	2,00,000	2,00,000
2	Standard Deduction	30,000	30,000	30,000
3	Taxable Salary	1,70,000	1,70,000	1,70,000
4	Tax at Present Rate	25,000	25,000	25,000
5	Rebate at Present Rate	15,000	15,000	10,500
6	Gross Tax Payable	10,000	10,000	14,500
7	Special Tax Relief on Sex	Nil	5,000	Nil
8	Net Tax Payable	10,000	5,000	14,500
9	%of Net Tax before SD	5.0%	2.5%	7.25%
10	% of Net Tax after SD	5.8%	2.9%	8.5%

Table 2
Benefits Enjoyed by the Families of Double Earnings (DE) and Single Earnings(SE)

Sl. No.	*Particulars & Benefits*	*Family "X" Double Earnings (Rs.)*	*Family "Y" Single Earnings(Rs.)*
1	Total Income of the Family	4,00,000	4,00,000
2	Benefits Enjoyed		
(a)	Standard Deduction	60,000	30,000
(b)	Maximum Tax Free Limit	1,00,000	50,000
(c)	Rebate	30,000	10,500
(d)	Special Rebate on Tax	5,000	Nil
(e)	Savings/Investments	2,00,000	70,000
(f)	Interest on Savings @ 9%	Per Year 18,000	Per Year 6,300
(g)	Total Benefit on Spot	3,95,000	1,60,500
	% of Benefits on Total Income	98.75%	40.12%

	Every Year Future Benefit:	Rs. 18,000	Rs. 6,300
(h)	Tax Payable	15,000	14,500
(i)	% Tax on total inflow of cash into the family	3.75%	7.25%

Table 3

Comparative Assessment of DE Group and SE Group in Two Families

Sl No.	*Particulars*	*Family X DE Group*	*Family Y SE Group*	*Revenue to Govt. (Rs.)*
1	Number of Members Husband, Wife and Three Children	05	05	---
2	Number of Earning Members	02 Husband & Wife	01 Husband	---
3	Income Per Head @ Rs. 200000	4,00,000	2,00,000	---
4	Standard Deduction @ Rs.30,000 (At Present Structure - APS)	60,000	30,000	---
5	Savings for the Tax Rebate- APS	2,00,000	70,000	---
6	Tax Rebate General- APS	30,000	10,500	---
7	Tax Rebate for Female- APS	5,000	---	---
8	Total Tax Rebate- APS	35,000	10,500	---
9	Net Tax (APS)	15,000 10,000+ 5,000	14,500	29,500

Table 4

Assessment of DE Group Family "N" and SE Group Family "R" Whose inflow of the Cash is Rs. 4,00,000 As per the Present way of Assessment

S.No.	*Particulars*	*Family N DE Group*	*Family R SE Group*	*Revenue to Govt. (Rs.)*
1	Number of Members Husband, Wife and Three Children	05	05	---
2	Number of Earning Members	02 Husband & Wife	01 Husband Only	----
3	Income Per Head @ Rs. 200000 for Family N and Rs. 400000 for Family R	4,00,000	4,00,000	----
4	Standard Deduction @ Rs.30,000 (At Present Structure - APS)	60,000	30,000	----
5	Savings for the Tax Rebate- APS	2,00,000	1,00,000	----
6	Tax Rebate General- APS	30,000	15,000	----

S.No.	Particulars	Family N DE Group	Family R SE Group	Revenue to Govt. (Rs.)
7	Tax Rebate for Female- APS	5,000	----	----
8	Total Tax Rebate- APS	35,000	15,000	-----
9	Net Tax (APS)	15,000 10,000+ 5000	70,000	85,000
10	% of Net Tax on Income after S.D	4.4%	18.9%	
11	% of Net Tax on Income before S.D	3.75%	17.5%	

Table 5

Comparative Assessment of Income on the basis of the Suggested Concept of Family Assessment

Sl. No.	Particulars	Family N DE Group	Family RSE Group	Revenue to Govt. (Rs.)
1	Number of Members Husband, Wife and Three Children	05	05	---
2	Number of Earning Members	02 Husband & Wife	01 Husband	----
3	Income Per Head @ Rs. 200000	4,00,000	4,00,000	----
4	Standard Deduction @ Rs.30,000 rate At Present Structure - APS	50,000	30,000	----
5	Savings for the Tax Rebate- APS	1,00,000	1,00,000	----
6	Tax Rebate General- APS	15,000	15,000	----
7	Tax Rebate for Female- APS	----	----	----
8	Total Tax Rebate- APS	15,000	15,000	-----
9	Net Tax (APS)	64,000	70,000	1,34,000
10	% of Net Tax on Income after S.D	18.3%	18.9%	
11	% of Net Tax on Income before S.I	21.0%	17.5%	

Analysation

With the help of the above table the present tax structure is analysed here. Table 03 gives the comparative assessment of Individuals in the Family X and in the Family Y on the basis of individual assessment. Family X and Family Y, both are equal in family size, in the expenditure range and in social obligations. In family Y only the husband goes for Job i.e. only the husband is able to go for job due to the unemployment problems whereas in family X both husband and wife go for job. Here the assumption is that all Mr. A, Mrs.B of family X and Mr. C of the family Y get the same amount of salary/income say Rs. 2,00,000 p.a. If they are assessed individually:

Mr. A has to pay a tax of	Rs. 10,000	
Mrs. B has to pay a tax of	Rs. 5,000	Rs. 15,000
Mr. C has to pay tax of		Rs. 14,500
The Tax revenue to the Government		Rs. 29,500

It is already mentioned the benefits enjoyed by the family X. But the contradiction here is that the provisions of the Income Tax seem to be partial incase of the family with one person going for job. Because a family (DE Group) which is getting Rs. 4,00,000 as its income pays only Rs. 15,000 (Just 3.75%)as tax where as a family (SE Group) which is getting Rs. 2,00,000 as its income pays Rs.14,500 (7.25%). So the author feels that there is no Justice.

Now the Table 04 gives the comparative assessment of the Family X consisting of husband Mr. A and wife Mrs. B and another family Z consisting of husband Mr. D and wife Mrs. E. Here is also in family Z only one person i.e. husband Mr. D goes for but he earns Rs. 4,00,000 p.a. Family wise, these two families get the same amount of inflow of cash i.e the same income. But, if they are assessed for tax as per the present structure individually,

Mr. A has to pay a tax of	Rs. 10,000	
Mrs. B has to pay a tax of	Rs. 5,000	Rs. 15,000
Mr. D has to pay tax of		Rs. 70,000
The Tax revenue to the Government		Rs. 85,000

It is already mentioned the benefits enjoyed by the family "X". But the contradiction here is that the provisions of the Income Tax seem to be partial at high level incase of the family "Z" also with one person going for job. Because a family "X" (DE Group) which is getting Rs. 4,00,000 as its income pays only Rs. 15,000 (Just3.75%)as tax where as a family "Z" (SE Group) which is also getting Rs. 4,00,000 as its income pays Rs.70,000 (17.5%). So the author feels that there is no Justice in this case also.

One has to seriously think that one man earns Rs. 4,00,000 and he helps rather is asked to help the government resource by contributing Rs. 70,000 whereas two persons earn the same amount but they are asked to pay only Rs. 15,000. Such a long and vast injustice require justice. The family X with DE Group by enjoying a lot of qualitative and quantitative benefits from the government and by creating heavy social imbalance pays very less tax. Hence the author proposes the new concept to be introduced into the Tax Policy and the Tax Structure in the name of the Tax

Reform. The author is ready to clarify the doubts of anybody as far as the new concept of Family assessment is concerned. Hence by comparing the family X (DE Group) and family Z (SE Group) an assessment has been made at the present rates but on the basis of the newly proposed Concept of Family Assessment and presented in Table 05. Here the family X is given an additional benefit of Standard Deduction i.e. Rs. 50,000. Total cash inflow into the families in the name of income is taken for the calculation. As such:

Family X will have to pay a tax of	Rs. 64,000
Family Z will have to pay a tax of	Rs. 70,000
The government will get revenue	Rs.134,000

Justification

1. The Concept of Family Assessment is a newly proposed suggestive Assessment.
2. Families with SE Group are not all affected.
3. Families with DE Group contribute more to the Public Revenue on the basis of More Income More Tax and vice versa.
4. It is a type of progressive tax suggestion and progressive suggestion.
5. There may be strong criticism from the side of the DE group. But if they think seriously about the welfare of our Country in all dimensions and go through this article, there will not be any problem to implement the newly proposed concept.
6. The Social Imbalances will be reduced and inequalities will be removed.
7. There are chances for the increasing employment opportunities in long run.
8. Standard Deduction for the Family Assessment (DE Group) is fixed at Rs. 50,000.
9. Strong Rules are to be made and they are to be managed very carefully and without partiality. As far as the disclosure of income is concerned all the employees should necessarily declare the required information. That is possible through the strict disciplinary actions and crystal clear manual rules.

Suggestions

Tax is necessary to meet all the government expenditure for the betterment of the public at large. Taxation must aim at the increasing the public revenue without making the tax payers tired. The Following suggestions are offered for the Tax Reform which is the need of the hour to our country.

1. Now the income tax is calculated on the basis of the individual income particularly in the salaried group, individuals are very much specific This is the major area requires reformation. Instead of calculating the income tax on the income of a person(individual), income tax is to be calculated on the income of the family (Husband and Wife). That is, instead of calculating the inflow of the cash/income to an individual's pocket as taxable income for the purpose of computing the tax, it is highly suggested that the inflow of the cash/income into the family is to be calculated as taxable income for the purpose of computation of income tax.

2. It is expected that there will be a lot of opposition and resistance from the side of the family wherein both the husband and wife are going for job . Hence, it is suggested that a combined standard deduction may be given to the newly proposed concept of Family Assessment. Hence, for the family assessment, a standard deduction of 40% or Rs. 50,000 whichever is less may be given and it is suggested so. As far as the tax rate is concerned, there should not be any change for the family assessment. Maximum Tax Free Limit, Tax Rebates, Tax Rates applicable for the individuals (i.e Single Earner Group) are to be made applicable to the family assessment also (i.e Double Earners Group). The officers or the employees have to sincerely declare the fact about the spouse. Suppressing the facts has to attract severe punishment. One should seriously think about this suggestion at the interest of the Nation. To some extent, this will help the government to solve the unemployment problem also.

3. By taking all the points in to consideration, it is suggested that maximum tax free limit may be raised from Rs. 50,000 to 80,000. The monetary limit of Standard Deduction may be increased from Rs.30,000 or 40 % to 40,000 or 40% whichever is less for the individuals i.e SE Group and Rs. 50,000 or 40% whichever is less for the family assessment i.e DE Group. That is, the Standard Deduction may be 40% of the Gross Salary or Rs. 40,000 whichever is less and (for the proposed family assessment .

4. The following Tax rates are suggested:

Income from (Rs.)			*Income to (Rs.)*	*Rate in %1.*
1.	Rs.	01	80,000	Nil
2.	Rs.	80,001	Rs. 1,00,000	10%
3.	Rs.	1,00,001	Rs. 2,50,000	20%

4.	Rs.	2,50,001	and above	30%
5.	Surcharge: -		NIL	

Here the income means, the Income from Salary after the Standard Deduction, after the set-off of the accrued interest on the House Building Advance as per the existing rule and after the deduction under chapter VI (as usual what is going at present)

Conclusion

The above suggestions and concept of the Family Assessment are to be placed before the balanced learned persons, impartial experts, experienced economists, Nation Loving Patriotic to elicit their valuable analysation and approval in the name of the seminar and discussions. Once if the tax policy/structure is constructed in the light of the above suggestions and if the Concept of Family Assessment is introduced in the name of Tax Reform and if it is managed properly, I am sure that the inequalities among the salaried group will be removed to some extent, unemployment problems will be solved to some extent, Savings and Investments will be increased considerably and the public finance will go up certainly which will raise the fiscal resources. Such Tax Reform will convert our Indian Economy from the word "Developing" into the word "Developed".

37

Computation of Tax Liability of Co-Operative Societies

Introduction

Indian Planning has relieved basically on cooperative movement for transforming the rural sector. This was initiated to translate the ideas of democratic, socialism, into action and was expected to transform the social and economic structure of rural INDIA. Since the economic structure of India had its roots in villages, cooperative movement was conceived as the ' Principles Means for Bringing about changes of Fundamental nature in the economy'. And was expected to "evolve a scheme of Cooperative community organisations which touches upon all aspects of life". Cooperative movement is the best formula to develop land and other resources and various services in the common interest, at all levels of nation.

Cooperative societies have made a significant contribution in the uplift of weaker sections of societys. Our constitution is wedded to a socialistic pattern of society, it is a part of the government policy to promote and encourage them. Therefore Co – operative Societies enjoy several concessions under Income Tax Act, 1961.

Meaning

The essence of co-operation is that the isolated and powerless individuals can, by combining with one another, achieve advantages available to the rich and the powerful so that they may advance not only materially but also morally. To quote, The International Labour Force, Co-operative means, "an association of persons usually of limited means, who have voluntarily joined together to achieve a common economic...

undertakings." Prof. Paul Lambert, a leading authority on cooperation states "a co-operative society is an enterprise formed and directed by an association of users, applying within itself the rules of democracy and directly intended to serve both its own members and community as a whole".

But according to Income Tax Act, 1961 under section 2(19), Co – operative Society means co- operative society registered under the Co-operative Societies Act, 1912 or under the any other law for the time being in force in any state for the registration of the co-operative societies.

Urban consumer's co-operative societies means according to Income Tax Act, 1961, a society for the benefit of a consumer within the limits of a municipal corporation, municipality, municipal committee, notified area committee, town area or cantonment Board.

Types of CO-Operatives

Since, the co-operatives are concerned in the moral and social uplift of a depressed or weak section of the society, they may be formed practically in any walk of life. But from the point of view of business there are eight types of co- operatives.

1. Consumer Co-Operative Societies

This is the oldest form of business organisation under cooperation. These societies are formed by ordinary people for obtaining their day-to-day requirements of goods at cheaper prices. These societies make their purchases in bulk from wholesalers at wholesale rates from manufacturers at factory cost and then sell them to members and non, members at market prices. The surplus earned will be distributed among members in the form of bonus.

2. Producers' Co- Operatives

These societies are voluntary associations of small producers formed with the object of eliminating the capitalist class from the system of industrial production. The main object is to enable small producers to face competition from large producers. Members of these societies either produces goods on their own an sell these to their society for marketing the same of the society.

3. Marketing Co-Operatives

Marketing co-operatives are formed to act ass Central Sales Agency for their members some for the marketing cooperatives are also performing other incidental functions.

4. Housing Co-Operatives

These are the associations of persons who are interested either in securing the membership of a house or obtaining accommodation at fair and reasonable rents. Through these societies, members can secure not only financial assistance but also the economics (advantages) of purchase of building materials in bulk. The membership is open to all those who are interested in securing housing accommodation as well as to those who are ready to deposit money with the society for interest.

5. Credit Co-operatives

This refers the voluntary association of people with moderate means formed with the objects of extending financial accommodation for developing the habit of thrift among them. The funds of these societies consist of share capital contributed by members. This society may show consideration in granting loans to the poor people. Generally, the loans may be granted only for production purposes for which it may or may not ask security.

6. Co- operative Farming Societies

These societies are formed with the object of achieving the benefits of large scale farming and maximizing agricultural output. Membership is generally confined to the farmers including those owning land and those who merely till the land.

7. Processing Co-Operatives

These are generally set up in rural areas with the object of processing certain raw materials produced by agriculturalists for supply to industries, e.g., Co- operatives fro processing sugarcane, cotton, paddy, oilseeds etc.

8. Labour and Construction Co-operatives

The chief object of such societies is to progressively diminish the importance of contactors. These cooperatives consist of unskilled or semi-skilled workers as members organised in rural areas for carrying out irrigation and other purposes.

Assessment or Computation of Tax

The total income of co-operative societies is computed in the manner provided for any other Assessee/ Section 80 P of Income Tax Act 1961 provides for certain deductions to be made in computing the total income of a co- operative society.

Section 80 P (I) runs as income tax is not payable by a co-operative society in respect of certain incomes though they shall fork part of Gross Total Income of the society, as follows:

a. According to Section 80 P(2) (a) of income tax act 1961, a co-operative society engaged in some activities, the whole of the amount of profits and gains attributable to anyone or more activities shall be deducted. Specified activities include: -

(i) The business of banking or providing credit facilities to its members
(ii) A cottage industry
(iii) The marketing of the agricultural; produce of its members
(iv) The purchase of agricultural implements, seeds, livestock or other articles intended for agriculture for the purpose of supplying them to its members
(v) The collective disposal of the labour of its members
(vi) The processing, without the aid of power, of the agricultural produce of its members
(vii) Fishing, or allied activities, i.e., catching, curing, storing processing and marketing of fish or the purchase of materials and equipments in connection therewith for the purpose of supplying them to its members.

The cooperative societies engaged in the activities V and VII of the above can avail the Section 80 P (2) (a) only when they restrict the voting to the following classes of its members only.

(i) The individuals who contribute their labour or who carryon the fishing or allied activities
(ii) The cooperative credit societies, which provide financial assistance to the society
(iii) The State Government

(b) Primary Society engaged in supplying milk, oilseeds, fruits, and vegetables raised or grown by its members to:

(i) A federal co-operative society, which engaged in the business of supplying in the above, said products
(ii) The government or a local authority
(iii) The government company or a corporation established by a state or central acts (Statutory Corporations).

According to Section 80 P (2) (b) of the income Tax Act 1961, the whole of the amount of profits and gains from such business shall be deducted.

(c) The cooperative Societies engaged in activities other than those specified in the above mentioned activities, the seduction will be allowed, as per section 80 P (2) ©, in respects of profits and gains attributable to such activities amounted to Rs. 20,000.00 or actual profits and gains whichever is less.

If the society is a consumers' Co-operative Society, than the deduction will be Rs. 40,000.00 or actual profits and gains which ever is less.

(d) IN case of every cooperatives society, in respect of any income by way of interest or dividend derived from its investment with any other Cooperative society, the whole of such income, as per Section 80 P (2) (d), is to be deducted.

(e) In case of every cooperative society, in respect of any income derived from the letting of the godowns or ware-houses fro storage, processing of facilitating the marketing of commodities, the whole of such income, as per section 80 P (2) (e), shall be deducted.

(f) In case of every Cooperative Society not being a housing society or in which Consumers' Society carrying on transport businesses a society engaged in the performance of any manufacturing operations with the aid of power where the Gross Total Income does not exceeds RS. 20,000.00, the amount of any income by the way of interest on securities under Section 18 of the Income Tax Act or any income from the house property under section 22 of the Income Tax Act shall be deductible from the Gross Total Income.

(g) Rebate or bonus allowed on the purchases made by the members of a consumers' cooperative stores should be allowed as deduction as per circular Number, P.171 dated 22-8-1973.

(h) If a new industrial undertakings is run by cooperative society, an amount equal to 6% p.a. on Capital employed shall be deducted as power the provision to section 80 J (2), for the first seven assessment years from the year when it started production.

(i) According to the Section 80 I, a tax holiday for a period of 10 years has been allowed to a cooperative society in respect of 20% of the profit and gains derived from a newly started industrial undertakings or a hotel. But this concession is available to other assessees only for a period of 8 years.

Rates of Income Tax

The total income of the cooperative societies shall be chargeable to tax at the rates as follows for the assessment year 1985-86.

Where the total income does not exceed Rs. 10,000 15% of the income

Where the total income exceeds Rs. 10,000 But less than Rs. 20,000	Rs. 1,500 plus 25% of the amount by which the total Income exceeds Rs. 10,000

Where the total income exceeds Rs. 20,000 Rs. 4,000 plus 40% of the amount by which the total income exceeds Rs. 20,000 The amount of income tax computed at he aforesaid rate shall be increased by a surcharge calculated at the rate of 12% of income tax so calculated. Surcharge will not be charged with effect from assessment year 1986-87.

38

Management of Post-Tsunami Problems

Introduction

Twenty Sixth 26th December 2004 was a thick red letter day in the history of countries under Asian continents and so the case in Andaman and Nicobar islands. Yes, it was very terrible day started with sunrise by shaking the base. People were threatened terribly by dangerous waves named as Tsunami with roaring sound by taking the lives of the people and by leaving permanent sorrows, sufferings and adverse panic situation. The Earthquake and Tsunami have disturbed the major portions of Andaman and Nicobar islands, by leaving the permanent fear and stress in the minds of inhabitants of Andaman and Nicobar Islands as well as the tourists.

Present Problem

At present, the people of Andaman and Nicobar islands are totally in the state of confusion. Once in every day, there is jerking. Sometimes the jerking was intolerably strong which has been increasing the blood pressure of the people and the children. Everybody feels, at present, that they have some sort of giddiness, which is more or less like seasickness at the tune of sailing. People fear that the sea level may increase. The seawater may come to their residence and there may be heavy jerking. Almost all the people sleep outside their house during night hours. They are totally worried with confused-state of mind. As a result, the students do not study, could not concentrate, they fear even to go to their study-room inside the house. The parents fear to send their children to school due to innumerable crackings and less infrastructural facilities to escape from their buildings.

Another peculiar problem facing the Andaman and Nicobar islands is that the water level has increased after this tragedy of "earthquake" and 'Tsunami'. In some places, the water level has not come down to normal level where as in some other places, the sea has gone very far away from its previous level. People believe that this is due to only 'Tsunami'. This may be true to some extent, but the actual fact is that without bothering the carrying capacity of these islands, the southern parts of Andaman and Nicobar islands have been concentrated with the construction work especially in RCC constructions. As a result, the south has gone down to some extent compared to the north.

Major Problem

Now at present the main problem is that the inflow of the Sea Water into the Residential Areas and the Institutional Areas. Whatsoever be the impact on the basis of the Science and Arts, it is fact that the feelings and fear of the public, employees, students and children cannot be stopped. Now the major problem is that almost everyday during the high tide the sea water enters inside the residential and road areas of the Southern Part of these islands. In fact the residential areas constructed in the on-the-coastal areas have their house floor level at sea floor level.. Due to the unbalanced growth in the construction industry, high-scaled earthquake and the destruction role of tsunami waves, the Southern Parts of Islands have gone down and as a result the sea water comes inside. This will become a continue process of the Nature and the problems will be more during the rainy season.

Economic Complications

The Economy of the Andaman and Nicobar Islands is consisting of Agriculture, Industry, Trade and Commerce. These islands are grown at a heavy Cost of Investment. Due to this inflow of seawater into the residential areas, the occupants of the residential areas are vacating their residents and are going to high-level area. The government employees who were allotted quarters in the areas near the sea also vacate the quarters and applied for the change of accommodation. Because the seawater enters, the agriculture will be affected totally. There will be acute shortage for the local vegetables, original cow milk, etc.. Due to this seawater problem, the labourers have left the islands. Even the local labourers fear that the inflow of seawater may go to the level of tsunami and thereby they do not come for the work. The shop owners employ the available highly skilled labour at high wages. This activity will affect the general public since they have to make more payment as the price and service cost. Since the seawater comes inside, the transportation of the raw materials has become difficult and as a result the industrial activities are affected.

Since the government employees are not given the quarters as per their entitlement, they prefer the private accommodation by increasing heavy demand for the same. These situations will worse the market for accommodation. The rental rate will go up and a middle class man particularly the unemployed persons and private employees cannot think of going for the private accommodation due to the role of the government employees. The government employees will never bargain and will be ready to pay more due to their House Rent Allowance. If the government says to vacate all the quarters where the sea water comes, practically the government can not provide accommodation at this moment. So the government will have to make a huge amount in the name of the House Rent Allowance. The problem will be more to the government in the case of a family where both husband and wife are going for job since the two people will get HRA. Commerce and Economics points of view, the Administration has invested a huge amount in terms of lakhs in the construction of quarters, hospitals, schools, colleges, and other institutions. By keeping these areas vacant and vacated, paying the HRA will be a great loss to the government.

What to do now? & How to Manage ?

Now the possibility of utilising the quarters with the safe standard of living and with the assured confidence by avoiding the unnecessary payment of house rent allowance are to be seriously considered. The highly invested buildings, where the hospitals, offices, schools, colleges, complexes, and potential agricultural land, the industrial units with the symptoms of sickness etc., are to be saved. Every body must seriously think about how to save this green paradise. Tourism Industry should be rejuvenated.

Suggestions

The people, officers, employees, children, students, businessmen, service centres etc., who are really in trouble due to the overflow of Sea Water everyday during the high tide and particularly during the Full Moon Day and No Moon Day. This cannot be stopped unless systematic and constructive steps are taken. The sayings of the scientists and experts are true. The implementing authorities may take these problems on the preferential ground and must come forward to solve the problems. Few suggestions are given below. This is only the expression of ideas and so Rejecting or Accepting is upto the readers of this article.

1. Research Findings for any problem or problems may be taken very seriously and the necessary interpretation and analysation are to be made by the responsible persons by inviting the researcher. Subject to the Provisions of the Acts or Laws, possibility of savings and retaining the buildings and quarters is to be decisioned. At this moment the major work in our hand is to decide how to save the residential area, life of the people, huge investment on the quarters, safe movements and to provide standard living. Regarding the frequency of the Tsunami, as per the Experts view, it may occur after many decades. That part let us give to the experts and scientists.
2. Immediately a committee consisting of the Highly Qualified Engineers, Researchers, Area Councilors/ Village Pradhan, Officers etc., is to be formed to inspect the quality of the buildings and quarters. They may be requested to go to the institutional buildings, residential buildings, etc., and verify the suitability of the building for the safety living. After getting the reports from the committee, subject to the provisions of the law and acts, the quarter's buildings are to be allotted to the employees as per their entitlement.
3. A careful analysis gives a result that the Sea Require Space for its routine day to day business. When it is blocked, it started overflowing and coming into the residential areas. So what we have to do at this moment is to return the space to the Sea. Otherwise, the Sea will take automatically at the cost our lives. So it is the high time to make a systematic design to give space to Sea. Experts' opinions are to be drawn without any politics for the whole island. A model for the Junglighat Area is given below for the deep thinking of the experts, general public, learned persons, critics and the authorities responsible for the development of these islands.
4. During Full Moon Day and No Moon Day, the Sea Water Enters into the residential area particularly the Quarters Side. The roads are full of water which goes upto 1-3 feet, the quarters upto2-3 feet and shops 2-4 feet etc. No one can travel by that time, people can not walk around, people fear what will be next in the Agenda of the Nature, people can not sleep, children can not study, and so on. The Normal Life of the People gets disturbed. So it is suggested that a Safe Retaining Wall at a width of 3 feet, depth of 15 feet (4 feet above the Civil Road Floor 5 Feet above the Sea Floor and 6 feet below the Sea Floor –as foundation). The Wall Should start from high beam area of the Murtha Khadi, and run just side by the road by keeping the Park area inside the sea to the proposed wall. The wall has to be

extended upto the Road where the Durga Puja Ground Ends. By leaving the present road to the ground side, from that angle at 90 degree same size Wall is to be constructed to the point adjoining the present Vijay Bhag retaining wall and that wall should go by rounding the Dairyform Base Area to the possible extent as per the advise of the Experts. The quarters and private properties covered by these catchments are to be immediately vacated. Atleast one meter depth, the sand is to be removed from the sea and they must be put on the road with a view to raise the height of the road as per the advise of the committee.

5. The Private Parties, Quarters, encroachment portion of the sea area are to be totally vacated. Sand is to be removed at a depth of 0ne meter from the Retaining Wall Covered Area in such a way the sea will come inside during the high-tide time so that the there would not be over flow of Sea Water into the Residential Area. All the huge amount invested quarters, hospital, etc. can be saved. The problems will be solved permanently. The cost of this proposed project will not be that much when comparing the problems of overflow of the seawater which will arise in future if this project is not considered.

6. The Same manner, south point college and girls' high school area are to be developed with a view to save the buildings from the Sea Water. The retaining wall, which runs in front of the college, should continue towards the east and west straight. Towards east the wall may touch the turning of the Alai Kaddal Iyyanar Temple by leaving the portion for the sea. Towards west at 180 Degree should touch Aberdeen Bazaar Post Office Turn by replacing the Marina Park to the right hand side of the road on the Gymkana Ground with the available space. The bent road side area near the college and the Marina Park Area to the extent possible are to be given to the Sea without disturbing the water sports complex.

7. A careful design is to be drawn without the meaningless talks of the tiro-tyros by leaving the politics. The sand to be removed from the proposed area for the Sea is to be put in a low level area to rise the heights.

8. Next the educational institutions are to be concentrated. The JNRM is in a very bad shape. Water comes inside the college and the near the classrooms and produces untolerable smell. Subject to the Provisions of the Acts & Laws, by retaining the RCC building, all the broken old timber based sheds are to be totally removed. Only the

Science Courses may be conducted in the RCC Structure. The College for Arts may be opened in Dairy Farm Area. The College for Commerce may be opened in the Delanipur Area. A suitable Management System Design is to be constructed carefully.

9. The possibility of shifting the educational institutions on the basis of the cost benefit analysis and due to the effect of overflow of the sea water into the residential area and institutional areas is to be considered by taking the present situation. The Mayabunder College may be shifted to Rangat. Polytechnic I may be shifted to High Level Area of the Bambooflat and the Polytechnic II may be shifted to Mayabunder Area where the Govt. College is run at present. The Girls High School may be shifted to the Polytechnic Building in Dollygunj with the fully protected Bus Service for the Girl Students.
10. Mangrove Forests will solve major problems. Mangrove Forests are to be developed nearby the sea shore after having a thorough discussion with the related experts with research oriented academic professors.

Conclusion

Giving suggestions is very easy to every one. But the how much difficulty in implementing a particular suggestion is known only to the people who are involved in the execution work. At the same time, we can not simply neglect the important responsibilities of taking decisions and implementing. The highly invested buildings are to be saved, unnecessary payments are to be stopped, the quarters are to be occupied, institutions are to be functioned, market conditions are to be brought under normal situation, agricultural land must get its fertility power. So we have to make a systematic design so that the sea water will not come inside the residential area. Now the sea requires its space which we have occupied from the sea few decades back. Now we have to return the same to the sea. This is the simple logic. If we do not return, the sea will automatically take its space at the cost of our lives. If a suitable strategy is made and a project designs for all the places of Andaman and Nicobar Islands are constructed in the light of the above suggestions, the residential areas may be saved, the quarters may be re-allotted after having a survey for repair, the fear in the minds of the public will go, a new look for the city will come, buildings can be saved, institutions can be utilised, the economic conditions will improve, we can see back the vegetables, small units will be recovered from the sickness and such improvements will again attracts the tourists to our ever green paradise. Please come let us all work for our union territory of Andaman and Nicobar Islands which has been giving Rotti for us.

PART V

CONCLUSION

Growth and Development are very important for every country. Social growth, political growth, cultural growth, industrial growth, trade growth and commerce growth are very essential for the development. The economic growth and development forms the basis for the above growths. The available resources are to be systematically exploited without damaging the eco system of the place. The potentiality of the trade, commerce and industry and marketing of the goods and services is to be explored. Infrastructural facilities are another important aspect, which are to be made available. Functions, festivals and celebrations are to be encouraged i.e. they must go on its normal way without the loss of any life of living beings (that the bali should not be given and the slaughter of the animals should not be in the functions and celebrations) so that the social growth and cultural growth can be seen.

The importance of savings, capital formation, investments for future, making provision for permanent income in future are to be well understood for the fiscal growth and development. Need for the strong primary, secondary and higher education and high level science and technology, innovation and inventions, reformation in the educational and examination system, tax structure, reduced transport cost tariff is to be really felt. Need for the foreign exchange through the export and global trade through the quality goods and services are to be realized in true sense. To bring the above symptoms as the situation and status position, every country has been trying their level best since quite a long time. But the result is unsuccessful though not failure.

The main reasons for this are poor planning, inefficient organisation, defective communication, baseless direction, system-less functions, less qualified staffing, meaningless control, absence of coordination and careless budgeting. The people who placed on the responsible position are supposed to plan each and every activity of the system of the management. The drawbacks, failure, carelessness, the quality of taking everything light in the name of positive approach on negative thinkings and happenings, inefficiency, un-productivity on the part of the officers on the responsible position, will definitely make the whole investment of funds; investment of energy, productive time, potential hard work and dedicatedness of the efficient people; and the inserted resources etc. to the status of failure along with irrecoverable loss, irrepairable damages, irredeemable investment and unsolvable problems to the country or nation as a whole. Hence in actual sense, the growth can not be seen. So the systematic planning is the only remedy.

Planning means deciding in advance. Here deciding in advance means deciding for decision by analyzing the Pros and cons, merits and demerits, advantages and disadvantages, favorable and adverseness, possible criticisms, benefits and problems. It is not a case that based on thinking something in dreams, compulsion by a group of people having vested interested, and pressure from the political parties, of taking decision and implementing for the result of failure. The quantum of getting success and bringing the meaningful growth and development fully depends upon the extent of effective deciding in advance and taking decision. This is called planning. Hence, planning plays a vital role in the process of economic growth and development. Though the management is focused on the environmental factors, the systematic planning can solve the related problems and save the organisation as the ozone layer saves living beings on the earth.

By taking the planning as the basic function for the economic growth and development, the factors and determinants are identified. They are Business Related Factors (BRF) namely consumers, entrepreneurs, trade, commerce and industry and tourism, Education Related Factors (ERF) namely higher education including examination reformation, science and technology etc., and Problems Related Factors (PRF) namely corruption, unemployment, tax reforms, and tsunami etc

The consumers are the eyes of the business. Entrepreneur is the essence of the business unit because, he bears the risks, combines the other factors and performs the functions, he innovates the new things, undertakes the venture business activities and mixes the 5 Ms, namely Money, Materials, Mechanisms, Men, Machines. While planning, this factor of the growth and development has been given very limited importance. So both the consumers and the entrepreneurs base and foundation of the Economic Growth and Development

Trade, Commerce including Tourism and Industry play an important role in the economy of any country. Growth of these sectors is the parameter to measure the economic development in a country particularly developing country like that of India. Further, the trade, commerce including tourism and industry offer ever-widening employment opportunities. Besides generating income and employment opportunities, the development of trade, commerce and industry gives an impetus to social relationships.

Education is a unique feature that plays the most dominant role in the life and evaluation of mankind and thereby creates a real human resource (real asset). The economic development of the country depends fully upon such real assets. Hence, education – Primary, middle, secondary, higher secondary, college plays a vital role in shaping, sharpening and refining the personality of the person. Higher education provides a proper solution to each problem of human beings, trade, commerce, industry, social, spiritual, culture, political, agriculture, administration, services, and the quality of overall environment.. Education, by the curriculum wise, is divided in the Science Education, Technical Education, Arts Education and Commerce Education. Commerce includes Finance (Banking), Transport, Insurance, Storage, and Advertisement and Publicity. All activities and transactions such as the how to manage, how to prepare accounts, how to bring the relations with the other factors, how to plan, how to organise, how to direct, how to select the personnel, how to control, how to coordinate, how to communicate, how to report and how to budget and estimate etc., related to the Banking, Transport, Insurance, Storage, Advertisements and Publicity are all called commerce activities and the education about such actions and transactions is called Commerce Education which is the basis for the growth and development.

Science and Technology helps the entrepreneurs to go "International". So the entrepreneurs must have the art and science of the business and the activities of the business and management of the units. Innovation is the cover term for the activities of bringing new ideas and invention is the cover term for the activities of bringing something solidly in a physical shape to the world.

The major problem in the process of smooth growth is the corruption, which means the "abuse of public office for private gain" and unemployment is the real problem of a country. It creates inequalities of income, economic imbalance and frustration in the minds of the young educated youth who are going to be the tomorrow's administrators. The unemployment problem kills the family as a whole. It tempts the unemployed youths (may be of the real human resource) to commit suicides for the want of every day's bread and social prestige. Due to this unemployment problem, the youngsters will be attracted towards the unwanted and anti-national elements. The unemployment problem is a great obstacle to the economic growth and development.

At present the tax structure is very complicated with the absence of natural base and justice. At micro level it is, no doubt, one sided. It is clearly mentioned in the principles of taxation that the Tax Structure/Policy should aim at the increase the resources, reduction of the inequalities, increase the savings and investments and to control the government expenditure. All these principles must be present in the Tax Policy. But the present Tax Structure is not of a full-fledged one. So there is an absolute need for the Tax Reform for the uninterrupted growth and development.

Due to the Tsunami destructive waves, the students do not study, could not concentrate, they fear even to go to their study-room inside the house. This present state of fear is to be totally avoided through a balanced, systematic and corruption-less management of post tsunami problems for the rehabilitation of the people of the affected areas which is the pre requisite for the growth and development.

It is easy to give suggestions, to recommend schemes etc. but the feasibility of their implementation should be taken into consideration particularly from the point of view of finance. By and large, all suggestions, made above, are economically viable and feasible and worth trying. The A & N islands has vast potential resources to be exploited for the economic growth and development with the geographical disadvantage of distance from the mainland of India with heavy increasing rate of population. It is upto the planners and the A & N Administration, Govt. of India, Development authorities to provide more infrastructural facilities so that the economic sector including tourism industry will grow to a greater extent which will contribute to the development of Indian Economy.

Once the impediments in the path of the Planning for Growth and Development are removed and if the effective strategies, programmes, policies, and rules are framed in the light of the suggestions given in each articles, and the same are carefully implemented, executed and monitored, by the dedicated and hardworking officers the economic growth will definitely emerge which will take any region, area or the country as a whole to the economic development.

Bibliography

I–Books

1. A&N ADMINISTRATION. , 1970-2004. *Basic Statistics*, Port Blair.
2. AMBASHT, N. K., 1970. *Critical Study of Tribal Education* .New Delhi: S. Chand & Co.
3. AWARADI, S. A., 1990. *Computerised Master Plan* (1991-2021). Port Blair: A & N Administration.
4. BASU, B.K., 1990. *The Onge Negrito Hunter-gatherers of Little Andaman*. Calcutta: Seagull Books.
5. BASU, BADA KUMAR. , 1990. The *A & N Islands Tribal Series*. Calcutta: Seagull Books.
6. BONNINGTON, M. C. C., 1932. *Census of India-1931* Andaman and Nicobar Islands. Calcutta: Superintendent Government Printing.
7. BROWN RADCLIFF, A.R., 1922. *The Andaman Islanders*. London: Weidenfeld & Nicolson.
8. BROWN, FRANCIS J., 1961. *Educational Sociology (N.J)*. Tokyo: Charles E. Tuttle Company: (2nd Edition).
9. CHAK, B.L., 1967. *Andaman and Nicobar Islands*, Ministry of Information and Broadcasting .New Delhi: Government of India.
10. CIPRIANI, L., 1966. *The Andaman Islanders*. London: Weidenfeld & Nicolson.
11. DAGAR, J.C., MONGIA A.D. AND BANDAPADHYAY A.K., 1991. *Mangroves of Andaman and Nicobar Islands*. New Delhi: Oxford and /Bit Publication Co.
12. DAS GUPTA, N.K., 1963. *Problems of Tribal Education and the Santhals*. New Delhi: Bharatiya Adimjati Sevak Sangh:
13. DAS, H. H. & DAS, SUSMITA.,1988. *The National Movement in India*. New Delhi: Renaissance Publishing House.
14. DAS, S.T., 1982. *The Andaman and Nicobar Islands*. New Delhi: Sagar Publishers.

15. DOSHI, S.L., 1978. *Processes of Tribal Unification and Integration*. New Delhi: Concept Publishing Company:

16. DURKHEIM, EMILE.,1956. *Education and Sociology (translated)*, Glencoe. New York: Free and Faber Ltd:

17. EISANSTADI, S.N., 1975. *Modern Political Theory*. New Delhi: Vikas Publishing House.

18. EVERMETT, F. H., 1971. *How Economic Growth Begins* – A Theory of Social Change in Finkle J.L & Richard W.Galblic, Political Development and Social Change. John Wee lay: Place.

19. GHOSH, A. K., 1955. *Nicobarese*: Andaman and Nicobar Islands, Census of India 1950.Delhi: Manager of publications.

20. GUPTA, B., 1976.*Andaman: The Land of Primitives*. Calcutta: Jinjnasa Publications.

21. GUPTA, B., 1976. *Andaman: The Land of Primitives*.Calcutta: Jinjnasa Publications.

22. HADDON,A.C.,1924. *The Races of Man and their Distribution*. London: Milner & Co.

23. HAMBLY, W.D., 1960. *Origin of Education Among Primitive Peoples*. New York: The Mac Millan Co.

24. HELSER, ALBERT.D.,1934. *Education of Primitive People*. New York: Fleming H. Ravel.

25. HERTE E., 1923. *Stories from Car Nicobar- Census of India*(1921). Calcutta.: Manager of Publications.

26. JUSTIN, A., 1990. The *Nicobarese*. Calcutta: Anthropological Survey of India.

27. KLOSS, C.B., 1903. *In the Andaman and Nicobar Islands*. London: John Murray (Indian reprint 1971).

28. KOPPIKAR, G.K., 1956. *The Education of Adivasi*. Delhi: Manager of Publications.

29. KUPPUSWAMY, B., 1975. *Social change in India*. Delhi: Vikas Publishing House.

30. LOWIS, R.F., 1923. *Census of India*, Andaman and Nicobar Islands (1921). Calcutta: Manager of Publications.

31. LOWIS, R.F., 1923. *Census of India, Andaman and Nicobar Islands* (1921). Calcutta: Manager of Publications.

32. MAJUMDAR, D. N. & T. N. MADAN.,1956. *An Introduction to Social Anthropology*. Bombay: Asia Publishing House.

33. MAJUMDAR, D.N., 1951. *Races and Culture of India*. Lucknow: Universal Publishers.

34. MAJUMDAR, D.N.,1948. *Races and Culture in India*. Bombay: Asia Publishing House.

35. MAJUMDAR, R. C., 1975. *Penal Settlement in Andamans*. Delhi: Ministry of Education.

36. MALHOTRA,O.P., 1986. *Tribal Education in A & N Islands*. New Delhi: S. Chand & Co.

37. MAN, E. H., 1883. *The Aboriginal Inhabitants of Andaman Islands*. London: Indian reprint Delhi, Sanskaran Prakasan.

38. MAN, E.H., 1923. *Nicobar Islands and Their People*. England: Royal Anthropological Institute.

39. MANN, R .S., 1979. *The Bay Islanders*. Calcutta: Institute of social research and Applied Anthropology.

40. MATHUR, K.K.,1967. *Nicobar Islands*. Delhi: Sterling Publishers (p) Ltd.

41. MATHUR, L.P., 1968. *History of The Andaman and Nicobar Islands*. Delhi: Sterling Publishers (P) Ltd.

42. MATHUR, L.P., 1968. *History of The Andaman and Nicobar Islands*. Delhi: Sterling Publishers (P) Ltd.

43. MODAK, TARABI.,1962. *The Meadow School*. Delhi: Manager Govt. of India Press.

44. MOUAT, F.J., 1863. *Adventures and Researches among the Andaman and Nicobar Islands*. London: Hurts and Blackwell.

45. MOUNT FORT, G., 1988. *Rare Birds of the World*. London: Collins.

46. NAIK, T. B., 1969. *Impact of Education on the Bhils*, Cultural Change in the Tribal Life of Madhya Pradesh. New Delhi: Planning Commission.

47. PANDIT, T.N.,1990. *The Sentinalese*. Anthropological Survey of India, Calcutta.

48. PANIKKAR, K. M., 1971. *India and The Indian Ocean. Bombay*, George Allen and Unwin.

49. PORT MAN, M. V., 1899. *A history of our relations with Andamanese*. Calcutta: Superintendent of Govt. Printing Press.

50. RAJAVEL, N., 1998. *Tourism in Andaman and Nicobar Islands*. Delhi: Manas publication.

51. RAJAVEL, N., 2003. *Management of Higher Educational Institutions*, Delhi: New Century Publications.

52. RATHANIAH., 1977. *Sanctural Constraints in Tribal Education*. New Delhi: Sterling Publishers.

53. REDCLIFF BROWN, A.R., 1922. *The Andaman Islanders*. Illinois: The Free Press.

54. RICHARDSON, REV. C. HOHN.,1947. *The Car Nicobar under Japanese occupation* 1943-45(Car Nicobar).

55. RIZVI, S.N.H., 1990. *The Shompen: A vanishing Tribe of the Great Nicobar Island*. Calcutta: Seagull Books.

56. SALDANHA, C .J., 1989. *Andaman Nicobar and Lakshadeep*, An Environment Impact Assessment. New Delhi: Oxford and IBH Publishing Co, Pvt. Ltd.

57. SARKAR, S.S.,1951. *The Aboriginal Races if India*. Calcutta: Book land Private Ltd.

58. SARKAR.J.,1990. *The Jarawa*. Calcutta: Seagull Books.

59. SEN. P. K., 1964. *Land and People of the Andamans*. Calcutta: Post Graduate Mart

60. SHARMA, B .D., 1975. *Development of Small Tribal Communities-Theoretical Frame*. New Delhi, Ministry of Home Affairs.

61. SHARMA, S. P., 1991. *Census of India, Andaman and Nicobar Islards*. Port Blair Census Director.

62. SHYAM CHOWDHURY, N. K., 1977. *Social Structure of car Nicobar*. Calcutta: Anthropological Survey of India.

63. SPLINDER, GEORGE D., 1963. (Ed) *Education and Culture*. New York: Rinehart and Winston Inc.

64. SRIVASTAVA L.R.N.et.al.,1971. *Identification of Educational Problems of the Saora of Orissa*. New Delhi: NCERT.

65. SRIVASTAVA, L.R.N. et.al.,1971. *Developmental Needs of the Tribal People*. New Delhi: NCERT.

66. TAMTA, B.R., 1992. *Andaman and Nicobar Islands*. New Delhi: National Book Trust:

67. TEMPLE, R.C., 1901. *Nicobarese Reckoning-Census of India*. Delhi: Manager of Publications.

68. TEMPLE, R.C., 1903. *Authentic Cases of "Devil" Murders in the Car Nicobar*. Census of India 1901. Calcutta: Superintendent Government Printing.

69. VAIDYA, SURESH.,1960. *Islands of a Mary Gold Sun*. Delhi:Hindi Pocket Books (p) Ltd.

70. VIDYARTHI, L. P., 1960. *Indian Anthropology in Action*. Ranchi.

71. WHITEHEAD, GEORGE.,1924. *In the Nicobar Islands*. London: Seeley Services & Co., Ltd: .

II–Documents, Papers and Reports

1. ANTHROPOLOGICAL SURVEY OF INDIA.,1978. Calcutta: Andaman and Nicobar Islands Silver Jubilee Celebration 1951 – 76 (Souvenir).
2. CENSUS OF INDIA.,1941. Andaman and Nicobar Islands . Delhi :Govt. of India Publication.
3. KARUNAKARAN, G.,1962. Geology of the Andaman and Nicobar Islands, Andaman and Nicobar Information. Port Blair: A & N Administrations.
4. LOWIS R.F.,1912. Census of India(1911) Andaman and Nicobar Islands. Delhi: Manager of Publications.
5. MALLET, F.L.,1895. Volcanoes of Barren Islands, Records of Indian Geological Survey., 28: 28.
6. MAN, C. KING.,1869.Report on Nicobar Islands. Port Blair: A & N Administrations.
7. PLANNING COMMISSION .,1970.Team on Tribal Programme.Delhi: Govt. of India Publication.
8. REPORT ON THE ANDAMAN AND NICOBAR ISLANDS.,1942. Delhi: Govt. of India Publication.
9. RINK, P.H.,1847.Die Nicobar Insein. Records of Geological Survey of India., 77:105-153.
10. SHARMA, B.D.,1966.Jarawas, Census of India(1961)Port Blair: Census Director.
11. SINGH, S.,1952.Types of Human Adaptation in the Andamans. Geographical Review., 14(3).
12. STATISTICAL BUREAU.,1995. Basic Statistics of Andaman and Nicobar Islands. Port Blair: Statistical Bureau.
13. STEVENSON, C., 1971.Shompens of Great Nicobar. Census of India. Calcutta: Manager of Publications.
14. THAMPI, C.J.,1965.Soil Conservation Programme in Andaman and Nicobar Islands, Andaman and Nicobar Information. Port Blair: A & N Administration.
15. TRAYLOR, R.,1934.Native Life in the Andaman Islands. British Penal Settlement.
16. TURNBULL, C. M.,1968.Contemporary Societies, Hunting and Gathering. International Encyclopedia of Social Sciences(7).
17. VASU, D. N .,1953.Linguistic Introduction to Andamanese. Bulletin of Anthropological Survey of India 1(2): 55-70.

III–Journals and Magazines

1. ABDULAI, HUMAYUN. , 1966, More New Races Of Birds From The Andaman And Nicobar Islands, J. Of Bombay, Natural History Society., 63:420-422.
2. B.F.M.,1959. Possible Traces of Exogamous Divisions in the Nicobar Islands. Man., 9: 71-72.

3. BALKRISHNAN, N. B. AND NAIR, N. G., 1977. New Records of Plants from Andaman & Nicobar Islands, Indian Forestry. , 103: 638-640.

4. BALL, V., 1870. On the Language of Nicobarese. Records of Govt of India, 77: 258.

5. BARBE, R.P., 1846. Notices of the Nicobar Islands. J. Of Asiatic Society of Bengal.,15:344-367.

6. BASU, S.M., 1971. On Cannibalism Among Andaman Islanders. Vanyajati., 19(4): 136-137.

7. BHARGAB, O.P.,1956. Tribes of Andaman and Nicobar Islands. Forest Rangers College Magazine., 32: 85-93.

8. CHANDA, S., 1970. Customs related to birth and death among the Nicobarese. Modern Review. , 127(5): 333-334.

9. CHANDA, S., 1970.A traditional festival of Car Nicobarese Bulletin for the Anthropological Survey of India.,19(3-4): 247-257.

10. CHANDA, S., 1971. Devil Murder in Chowra: A Case Study. Folklore., 12(9): 328-332.

11. CHANDA, S., 1971. Economic Structure of Nicobarese Village in Chowra Island. Indian Journal of Social Work.,32(1):25-33.

12. CHANDA, S., 1972. Study of the Intra-Familiar Relationship among the Car Nicobarese. Indian Journal of Social Work.,32:109-116.

13. CHANDA,S.,1970. Car Nicobar Dweep Ke Ek Gram Ka Arthik Dhancha.Vanyajati .,18(4): 174-181.

14. CHANDA,S.,1970. Socio –Economic and Political Structure of Car Nicobar. Khadi Gramodyog : 625-634.

15. CHANDA,S.,1972. Some Traditional Festivals of Car Nicobar and their Significance. Bulletin of Cultural Research Institute., 9: 81-85.

16. CHANDA,S.,1977.Tribal Account In Transformation Of Car Nicobarese .Vanyajati .,25(4): 7-17.

17. CHATTERJEE, B.K.& DUTTAGUPTA, A., 1976. Customs Beliefs and Magical Rites of the Nicobarese. Mankind.,5:47.

18. CHATTERJEE, B.K.&BASU, D.N., 1953. Magico Religious Ceremony of the Nicobarese. Vanyajati.,1(2): 27-34.

19. DANDA,D.G.,1987.Little Andaman and The Onge Human Science.,36(1):66-91.

20. DANIEL LERNER.,1968.Encyclopedia of Social Science.,10:368.

21. EISENSTADI, S.N., 1954.African Age Groups. Africa, XXIV.

22. FONTANA,N.,1792.On the Nicobar Islands and the fruit of the Mellore. Asiatic Researches.,3:156

23. HAILEY, L.,1957. An African Survey, London.

24. HAMILTON,C.H.,1790..A Short Description of Nicobar. Delhi: Asiatic Researches.,2:339.

25. MAN, E.H., 1883. Aboriginal Inhabitants of Andaman Islands., 12:109-116

26. NAIR, B.R.,1979. Wild population of Areca and Cocoa in Andaman and Islands, Indian Journal of forests.,19: 350-362.

27. NAIR, N. G,1977. New records of Plants from Car Nicobar, Gobies., 4: 221.

28. NAIR, N.G, 1979 .Study on the Grass lands of Car Nicobar Island. Indian Jr. of Forestry.,2:254-260.

29. NAIR,N.G,1974. Happy Islanders of Nicobar.Mirror.,14(3):28-31.

30. OLDHAM, R. D.,1885. Note on the Geology of the Andaman Islands, Records of the Geological Survey of India.,18: pp135- 145.

31. OLDHAM, R. D.,1885. Note on the Geology of the Andaman Islands, Records of the Geological Survey of India.,18:135- 145.

32. PONDIT, T.N., 1976.Original inhabitants of the Andaman and Nicobar Islands, Yojana.,20(13):81-96.

33. RAJAVEL. N, 1996. How to Ensure Faster Growth, Industrial Herald Vol. 31(2) Jan.16-31, pp30-31

34. RAO, K.J.M., 1971. Andaman and Nicobar Islands- India in Miniature, Andaman and Nicobar Information: P-34.

35. REDDIAH, K., 1977.The coral reefs of the Andaman and Nicobar Islands, Rec. Zoological Survey of India.,72:315-324.

36. RINK, P. H., 1847. Die Nicobar Insein, Records of Geological Survey of India., 77: 105-153.

37. SACHIDANANDA.,1994. Tribal Education: New Prospective and challenges, Jr. of Indian Education.,19(6):30-35.

38. SINGH, H., 1988. Study Habits of Scheduled Tribe students in relation to their self-concept and level of aspiration, Jr. of Educational Research and Extension., 24(3): 67-174.

39. SUBBAKRISHNA,R AND JUSTIN,A.,1988. Hol-Chu: A Misnomer. 00-00-Human Science., 37(2): 187-189.

Index

T